Musculoskeletal Sonography
Technique, Anatomy, Semeiotics
and Pathological Findings in Rheumatic Diseases

Fabio **Martino**
Enzo **Silvestri**
Walter **Grassi**
Giacomo **Garlaschi**

Editors

Musculoskeletal Sonography

Technique, Anatomy,
Semeiotics and Pathological
Findings in Rheumatic Diseases

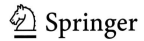 Springer

EDITORS

FABIO MARTINO
Chief of the Radiology Department
Giovanni XXIII-Policlinico Hospital
Bari, Italy

ENZO SILVESTRI
Department of Radiology
San Martino Hospital
Genoa, Italy

WALTER GRASSI
Professor of Rheumatology
Università Politecnica delle Marche
Chief of the Rheumatology Clinic
Jesi Medical Center
Ancona, Italy

GIACOMO GARLASCHI
Professor of Radiology
University of Genoa, Italy

Originally published as:
Ecografia dell'apparato osteoarticolare
Anatomia, semeiotica e quadri patologici
a cura di Fabio Martino, Enzo Silvestri, Walter Grassi, Giacomo Garlaschi
© Springer-Verlag Italia 2006

Translation by: see page XIII

Library of Congress Control Number: 2006934668

ISBN-10   88-470-0547-7 Springer Milan Berlin Heidelberg New York
ISBN-13   978-88-470-0547-1 Springer Milan Berlin Heidelberg New York

Springer is a part of Springer Science+Business Media
springer.com
© Springer-Verlag Italia 2007

Springer-Verlag Italia Srl, Via Decembrio 28, I-20137 Milano

Cover design: Simona Colombo, Milan, Italy
Typesetting: Graficando, Milan, Italy
Printing: Printer Trento Srl, Trento, Italy
Printed in Italy

Foreword to the Italian edition

It was with great pleasure that I accepted the invitation to introduce this publication, authored by my friends and colleagues Fabio Martino, Enzo Silvestri, Walter Grassi and Giacomo Garlaschi. The volume focuses on the impact of ultrasound in the musculoskeletal field, with particular reference to pathology in a rheumatological context. In fact, as noted, the social impact of **rheumatic diseases** *is significant, and an early clinical diagnosis is important, given that the incidence of these diseases is on the rise and that they often lead to highly disabling conditions. Increasingly sophisticated and advanced ultrasound techniques have allowed the definition of important initial aspects of the disease, concerning synovial involvement, with pannus formation and cartilaginous joint damage. Moreover, the subsequent and ever increasing use of contrastographic techniques has allowed acquisition of the clinically and therapeutically important parameters of* **objective evaluation** *(the degree of hyperemia and flow quality)* **of the active and quiescent phases of the chronic arthritis.***

The book is presented in three distinct sections: in the first (chapters 1-3), principal technological aspects and the multiple exam procedures are discussed, with the pertinent anatomy both under basal conditions and using the Doppler technique. The second section (chapters 4-5) represents, without doubt,

the most innovative and didactic work within the volume through its rigorous and precise analysis of ultrasound semiotics of the musculoskeletal apparatus and with its multiple descriptions of disease patterns. These are made more resonant through the use of excellent and carefully chosen iconography. This section is further enhanced with a description of the role of ultrasound in monitoring chronic inflammatory joint disease during therapy (chapter 6). Finally, the last section (chapter 7) deals in a prospective manner with some interesting applications of ultrasound in the therapeutic arena that, in the near future and upon further refinement, could represent a precious and irreplaceable complement to a therapeutic program that is becoming increasingly defined and essential.

In conclusion, the experience and impressive didactic talents of the authors are divulged by the lucid text, the precise and up-to-date bibliography and the painstakingly designed iconography. This book will certainly represent a useful and interesting travel companion for all specialists, demonstrating that the radiologist plays a role that is increasingly clinical and is not simply that of an anonymous arranger of images; no longer an extra, but a main player in the co-management of the complex and difficult world that is today considered the "Rheumatological planet".

Prof. Carlo Masciocchi
Director of Radiology Institute
University of L'Aquila, Italy

Foreword to the English edition

Musculoskeletal ultrasound has established itself as a highly versatile and precise imaging tool. In the beginning only a few enthusiasts sporadically applied ultrasound to musculoskeletal disorders, and it is only relatively recently that evidence has been gathered as to how valuable the technique can be in reliably making an accurate diagnosis. The continued development and application of new techniques that improve spatial soft tissue resolution will undoubtedly increase its future role.

It is therefore timely and indeed very welcome that the distinguished Editors of this book have put together the state-of-the-art knowledge on the application of ultrasound in rheumatology. The authors are highly respected and cover the global extent of the field bringing the reader up to date by discussing and analysing the various rheumatological pathological conditions.

The design of this work is very practical and reader-friendly. It is presented in a format which shows a great deal of editorial forward planning and execution. Technological issues and procedure principles are presented with the liberal use of illustrations whereby the reader pictorially knows immediately where and how the probe is placed on the area of interest, and is able to quickly correlate this with the expected sonographic appearances which are also anatomically well depicted in an atlas format. This section is designed for ease and quick reference as and when it is required. A normal anatomy section follows which is beautifully presented in a structured manner, and the same presentation structure is then used with some modification for the following section dealing with the sonographic features in pathological states. This section is without doubt outstanding living up to and clearly delivering the sonographic "doctrine of signs" (semeiotics). The illustrations are of the highest order all throughout leaving no ambiguity whatsoever. Where necessary and as if to show how far musculoskeletal ultrasound has come of age, correlation with MR images of the same patient and condition are provided. Having dealt with the pathological sonographic appearances of the various musculoskeletal tissues, the reader is then invited to a discussion on the application of ultrasound to the specific rheumatological conditions. The authors fairly define without bias the strength and weaknesses of ultrasound compared with other imaging modalities (predominantly MR imaging) as well as the value of colour and power Doppler techniques including the use of sonographic contrast agents. The last two sections although relatively short, outline the role of sonography in the therapeutic management of the diagnosed rheumatological conditions, both in monitoring the effects of therapy as well as a guide to the local administration of injection therapy.

On the one hand this book effortlessly presents a "how to do it" approach, while at the same time it delivers the evidence and advanced knowledge base of the relevant recent research concerning musculoskeletal ultrasound in rheumatology. It is therefore suitable to a wide audience from the novice embarking on providing a musculoskeletal ultrasound service, to the experienced musculoskeletal radiologist who wishes to add musculoskeletal ultrasound to his/her armamentarium.

Prof. Victor Cassar-Pullicino
Consultant Radiologist
The Robert Jones and Agnes Hunt Orthopaedic Hospital
Oswestry, United Kingdom

Table of contents

Chapter 5.   Pathological findings in rheumatic diseases

F. Martino, E. Silvestri, W. Grassi, G. Garlaschi, E. Filippucci,
C. Martinoli, G. Meenagh

Chapter 6.   **Ultrasonography and therapy monitoring**

F. Martino, E. Silvestri, W. Grassi, G. Garlaschi, E. Filippucci, G. Meenagh

Chapter 7.   **Ultrasound-guided procedures**

F. Martino, E. Silvestri, W. Grassi, G. Garlaschi, E. Filippucci, G. Meenagh

List of authors

Simone Banderali
Department of Radiology
University of Genoa, Italy

Bruno Bartolini
Department of Radiology
University of Genoa, Italy

Elviro Cesarano
Department of Radiology
University of Bari, Italy

Marco Falchi
Department of Radiology
San Martino Hospital
Genoa, Italy

Emilio Filippucci
Research Fellow in Rheumatology
University Politecnica delle Marche
Ancona, Italy

Alessandro Garlaschi
Department of Radiology
University of Genoa, Italy

Giacomo Garlaschi
Professor of Radiology
University of Genoa, Italy

Manuela Giglio
Department of Radiology
University of Genoa, Italy

Walter Grassi
Professor of Rheumatology
University Politecnica delle Marche
Chief of the Rheumatology Clinic
Jesi Medical Center
Ancona, Italy

Francesca Lacelli
Department of Radiology
University of Genoa, Italy

Fabio Martino
Chief of the Radiology Department
Giovanni XXIII-Policlinico Hospital
Bari, Italy

Carlo Martinoli
Associated Professor of Radiology
University of Genoa, Italy

Gary Meenagh
Research Fellow in Rheumatology
Musgrave Park Hospital
Belfast, UK

Alessandro Muda
Department of Radiology
San Martino Hospital
Genoa, Italy

Simona Parodi
Department of Radiology
University of Genoa, Italy

Laura Saitta
Department of Radiology
University of Genoa, Italy

Daria Schettini
Department of Radiology
University of Genoa, Italy

Luca Sconfienza
Department of Radiology
University of Genoa, Italy

Enzo Silvestri
Department of Radiology
San Martino Hospital
Genoa, Italy

Equipment and examination technique

1.1 Equipment

Ultrasound (US) is one of the best imaging techniques in musculoskeletal radiology because it is low in cost, has high spatial resolution, wide availability in hospitals, is well-tolerated by patients and is not biologically invasive, as it uses sound waves and non ionizing radiation, as in conventional radiology or computed tomography (CT). These features make ultrasound the ideal technique for the diagnosis and follow up of many pathologies and rheumatic syndromes and for the evaluation of the effects of therapy.

The high diagnostic value of ultrasound is strictly related both to the operator's knowledge of normal anatomy and to the effectiveness of ultrasound equipment to depict anatomical details (Fig. 1.1 a-c).

For this reason, the equipment and transducers' characteristics become very important when studying small and superficial structures, such as flexor and extensor tendons in fingers, which are very difficult to assess with other imaging techniques because of their superficial location.

The most recent generation of ultrasound equipment allows highly detailed depiction of structures located just a few millimeters from the transducer.

New generation transducers may reach very high frequencies (up to 20 MHz), that allow the evaluation of submillimetric structures, such as tendon pulleys (Fig. 1.2).

The availability of new multifrequency probes allows the simultaneous study of both superficial and deep structures, granting a good penetration of ultrasound waves through the tissues.

Assistance can be given by a silicone spacer or by a thick layer of gel when using old equipment (e.g. transducers under 10 MHz frequency).

Musculoskeletal sonography should be per-

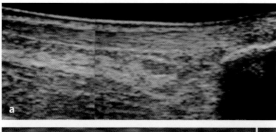
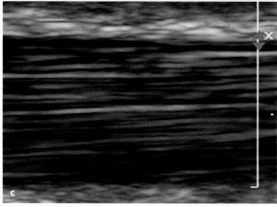
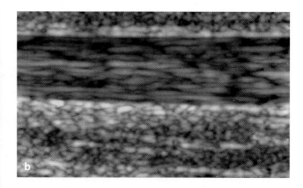

Fig. 1.1 a-c

Evolution in the resolution capability of tendon fibrillar echotexture. **a** Image obtained with ultrasound equipment from the early 90s: it is panoramic but has low spatial resolution. **b** Image obtained using ultrasound equipment from the late 90s with a good demonstration of the fibrillar echotexture. **c** Image obtained using the most recent generation of ultrasound equipment, showing great anatomical detail

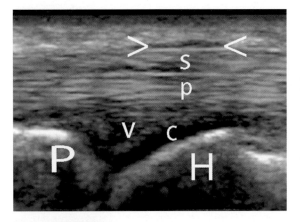

Fig. 1.2

High resolution longitudinal US scan of flexor digitorum communis: the *arrowheads* indicate the 1st reflection pulley. *H* = metacarpal head; *P* = proximal phalanx; *v* = volar plate; *c* = cartilage; *s* = flexor digitorum superficialis; *p* = flexor digitorum profundus

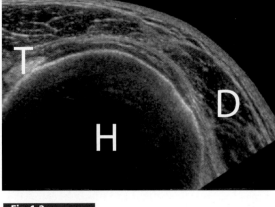

Fig. 1.3

EFV US scan of a shoulder that shows most of the humeral head (*H*), and the superficial tissues in a massive rotator cuff rupture. *T* = long head of biceps tendon; *D* = deltoid

formed with an excellent superficial definition (5 millimeters at least), because incorrect depiction of skin and subcutaneous tissue may cause artifacts and compromise the evaluation of clinical findings.

We suggest the use of ultrasound equipment with a very high-frequency transducer to assess the most superficial structures and a multifrequency transducer (about 7.5-12.5 MHz) to obtain a general evaluation of those deep musculoskeletal structures that cannot be easily studied with a very high frequency transducer.

When studying rheumatic diseases, it is mandatory to use ultrasound machines provided with a color and power Doppler module (low speed flows) to assess the synovial, tendinous or muscular inflammatory hyperemia [1-3]. Equally important is the set up for the use of contrast agents, which is particularly useful in the follow-up of the therapy [4, 5].

The visualization of images can be improved with different softwares, such as extended field of view (EFV), multi-planar bidimensional (MPR) and three-dimensional reconstruction (3D). These reconstruc-

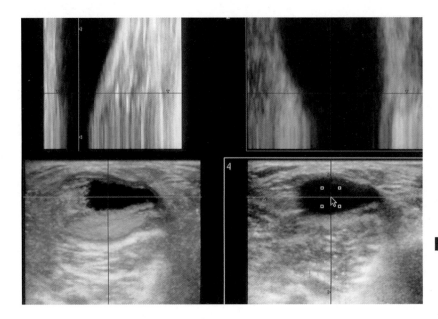

Fig. 1.4

Bidimensional MPR on three different spatial planes of a subfascial fluid collection following a muscular tear

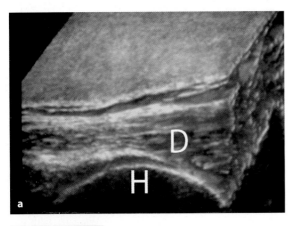
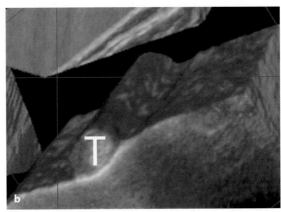

Fig. 1.5 a, b

a 3D rendered reconstruction of the shoulder showing the humeral head (*H*) and the deltoid muscle (*D*) with the superficial tissues. **b** 3D reconstruction of a shoulder with digital subtraction of superficial tissues. This allows the course of the long head of biceps tendon to be shown

tions do not improve the diagnostic level of the examination but make the images easy to interpret even by a non-radiologist. EFV allows the operator to 'build' a panoramic image of a wide anatomical region (such as a whole muscle or tendon) by simply gliding the probe along it. The images obtained are very easy to interpret [6,7]. Likewise, MPR and 3D allow panoramic reconstructions with a widened view of spatial planes to be created, as in CT and magnetic resonance (MR) (Figs. 1.4, 1.5 a, b). Nevertheless, image processing takes a long time to be completed and needs a perfect scanning technique to be effective.

1.2 Examination technique

Besides what has already been mentioned, it is compulsory to use some practical skills in order to avoid diagnostic pitfalls.

The patient must be positioned in a proper way to make the examination comfortable both for the patient and the operator, regardless of the examined anatomical region [8,9] (Fig. 1.6).

When studying the musculoskeletal system, particular attention must be paid to the angle of the ultrasound beam, which must be perfectly perpendicular to the examined structure. Otherwise, anisotropy-dependent artifacts (spatial asymmetry) may result in diagnostic errors, especially when studying fibrillar or fascicular structures such as tendons and nerves [10-13].

The anatomical regions where such artifacts

occur more frequently are some of the tendon entheses and the corresponding pre-insertional segments, where the tendon has a curvilinear course (supraspinatus, brachial biceps or Achilles tendon).

Longitudinal and transverse scans and sometimes also oblique and unconventional views must be performed in order to make a detailed assessment of the musculoskeletal structures.

Another essential feature of ultrasound that makes it unique among other imaging techniques, is that it permits dynamic assessment and therefore extracts important functional information. US is the only imaging technique that allows a direct

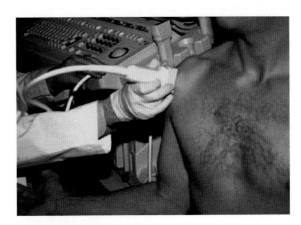

Fig. 1.6

Correct position of the patient for the assessment of the rotator cuff interaction between operator and patient through active, passive or resisted movement with the advantage of direct anatomic and functional visualization.

Moreover, the operator can take advantage of a comparative bilateral study to increase diagnostic confidence.

1.3 Artifacts

Artifacts result from the changes to which the ultrasound beam is subjected when passing through biological tissues. On the other hand, artifacts can also be due to the operator's using faulty scanning technique.

Operators must have a deep knowledge of the different types of artifacts because these can represent not only problem with image interpretation, but also an important source of diagnostic information.

In fact, while some artifacts reduce the diagnostic power of the scan (reverberation, mirror effect, partial volume, doubling, empty tendon artifact), there are others that can be extremely helpful in the differential diagnosis (posterior acoustic enhancement, acoustic shadowing, comet tail, ring down and rain artifacts) [8, 14].

Some artifacts can be avoided if the scan is performed in a proper way and the ultrasound equipment is properly set; others are caused by physical characteristics that cannot be changed but they must be understood in order to avoid diagnostic mistakes.

Posterior acoustic enhancement: an increase in echo intensity in tissues posterior to a fluid collection. It may not be detected when the fluid collection is small or spread over a large area (Fig. 1.7).

Acoustic shadowing: a weakening or absence of echoes posterior to a gas collection (high absorption of the beam), a bone surface (high reduction of the beam) or calcification (Fig. 1.8).

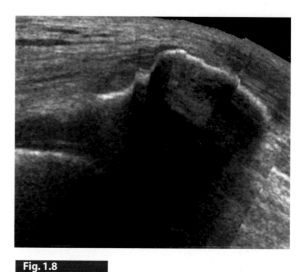

Fig. 1.8

Acoustic shadowing artifact on an EFV US scan of the patella

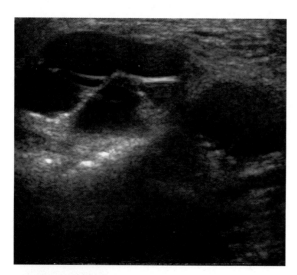

Fig. 1.7

Posterior acoustic enhancement artifact in a multiloculated cyst of Hoffa's fat pad

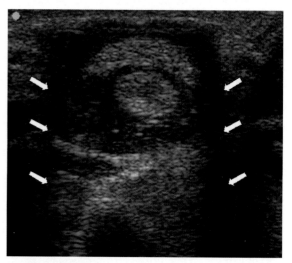

Fig. 1.9

Lateral acoustic shadowing artifact (*arrows*) in a tenosynovitis of flexor tendons of a finger

Lateral acoustic shadowing: it occurs when the ultrasound beam is tangential to tissues with different acoustic impedance. The wider the impedance difference, the more visible is the artifact (Fig. 1.9).

Rain effect: a reverberation artifact due to the gain curve. This is an important sign because it occurs when soft tissue overlies a fluid collection. It appears as a band of low-to-medium echoes lying parallel to the transducer and apparently arising from the soft tissue and moving down through the fluid (Fig. 1.10 a, b).

Reverberation artifact: due to its appearance, this artifact is also referred to as "ring-down artifact" and "comet tail artifact". It is caused by the reflection of the ultrasound beam several times back and forth between two nearby interfaces. The multiple echoes thus created reach the transducer before the next pulse transmission and produce multiple copies of the anatomy. Reverberation artifacts are commonly seen at soft tissue-to-gas/bone/metal interfaces (Fig. 1.11 a, b).

Mirror artifact: a duplication of the image occurring when the beam meets a highly-reflective interface causing reflection and reverberation phenomena.

Partial volume artifact: a noise that occurs when the ultrasound beam is wider than the scanned structure or the structure itself is just partially sectioned so that it is surrounded by tissues with different acoustic impedance. For example, if the beam sections a fluid collection that is narrower than the beam itself, a partial volume artifact will occur.

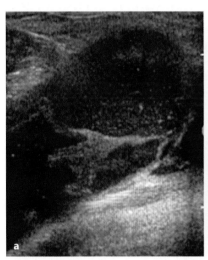 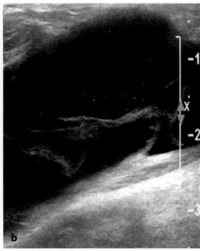

Fig. 1.10 a, b

a Rain effect artifact on the superficial layer of a multilocular Baker's cyst. **b** The artifact disappeared after the equipment was correctly set up

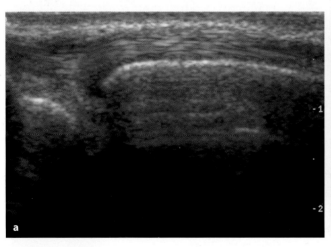 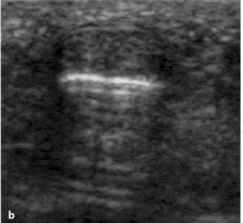

Fig. 1.11 a, b

Reverberation artifacts on a distal ulnar epiphysis (**a**) and on a phalanx (**b**)

Duplication and triplication: occurs when the ultrasound beam crosses two tissues with different acoustic impedance. It appears as a duplication or a triplication of the image when the structure measures less than one centimeter and as a deformation, enlargement or interruption when the object is larger.

Empty tendon artifact: a tendon appears homogeneously hypoechoic without the normal fibrillar echotexture (anisotropy) when using a sectional probe, because the progressive obliqueness of the beam highlights the anechoic appearance of the tendon. This artifact occurs when the ultrasound beam is not perpendicular to the tendon, on both longitudinal and axial scans, and can be avoided by tilting the beam almost perpendicular to the tendon (Fig. 1.12 a, b).

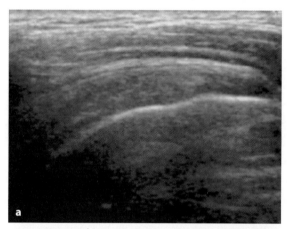

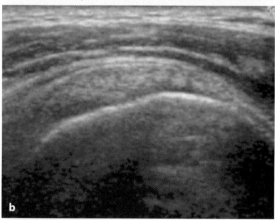

Fig. 1.12 a, b

a Anisotropy artifact on a tendon: insertion of supraspinatus with hypoechoic appearance of the tendon caused by incorrect insonation angle. **b** After a little adjustment of the transducer, the tendon appears normal

1.4 Doppler techniques

The Doppler effect is a physical phenomenon in which the frequency of a wave that hits a moving body undergoes a variation that is directly related to the speed of the body itself.

The difference between the outcoming and the incoming wave is called **Dn** (or *Doppler shift*).

The incoming wave has a higher frequency than the outcoming wave when the direction of the movement is towards the transducer while it has a lower frequency when the direction of the movement is opposite.

Therefore, the Doppler technique compares the two frequencies and measures the difference between them.

The equation that describes this phenomenon is
Dn = 2v f cos q/c
Where:
- *Dn* = is the difference between the incoming and outcoming wave;
- *v* = is the speed of the body;
- *f* = is the frequency of the outcoming wave;
- *q* = is the angle between the direction of the movement and the direction of the beam;
- *c* = is the speed of the beam in the tissue.

The transducer works like a normal ultrasound probe in all directions except one, selected by the operator. The Doppler scan is performed along this direction.

The operator sets the volume sampler within the vessel so that a speed and audio assessment of the flow can be performed. The obtained speeds are represented on a graph.

Moreover, with color Doppler, the obtained information can be represented as dot-by-dot color spots; each image is therefore the result of several processes: collection of data, encoding of B-mode and Doppler images and calculation of Doppler effect.

The flow inside the vessels appears as color spots with different features according to the examined vessel (Fig. 1.13 a, b).

The color scale that represents the flow can show three different parameters: direction (red: the flow goes in the direction of the probe; blue: the flow goes in the opposite direction), frequency and variance [8, 15].

There are some basic points to remember when using color Doppler:
- the color representation is strictly related to the shape of the vessel and of the transducer;

- there is no linear relationship between the speed values obtained from the color on the image and the values obtained from the spectrum analysis.

In addition, the angle of incidence of the beam is extremely important. Referring to the Doppler formula and calculating the value of cosine (cos 90° = 0), the optimum angle is < 60°, even though some difficulties in assessing the vessel can be encountered.

The introduction of power Doppler is fairly recent. It allows the detection of very slow flows and, thanks to the new techiques, their direction in relation to the transducer. Unfortunately, it is still not possible to obtain any semiquantitative color scales of the speed (Fig. 1.13 c, d).

Therefore, it is possible to sum up the characteristics of the Doppler effect as follows:

1. it allows to perform a qualitative analysis of flow signals, detecting their presence, direction and main characteristics;
2. it allows to perform a quantitative assessment of flow, measuring speed and blood capacity;
3. it allows to perform a semiquantitative evaluation, describing the spectrum of frequencies (i.e. width and systolic-diastolic modulation).

These Doppler techniques can be used to assess vessels in muscle thanks to the possibility of describing the caliber, the permeability and the presence of stenosis or pathological collateral circles (including malignant ones) [1].

Possible applications:
- inflammatory pathologies, where blood flow can be slackened to either a non-flow or a diastolic appearance (as in blood collection);

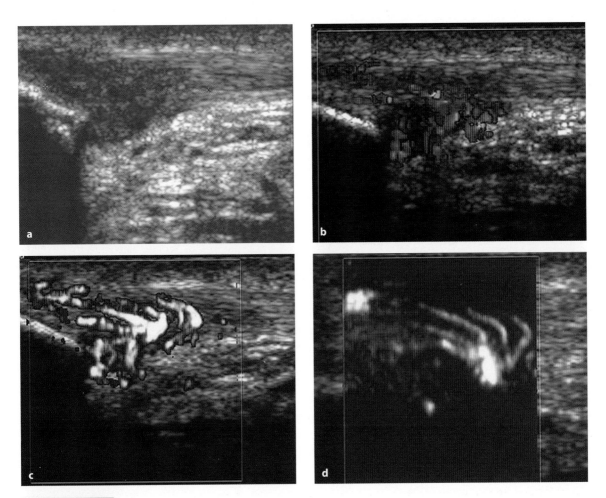

Fig. 1.13 a-d

Patellar tendon. **a** B-mode: focal hypoechoic area at the insertion caused by insertional tendinopathy. **b** Color Doppler: strong hyperemia in the same area. **c** Power Doppler shows a sharper definition of flows in the fibrillar structure. **d** Power Doppler mask: further increase of definition of the vascular pole and of its branches is shown

- traumatic pathologies, where it helps to understand the traumatic or surgical origin of hematomas that have an avascular appearance;
- malignant pathologies, giving the opportunity to characterize the lesion (even partially); in fact, benign lesions usually present regular vascularization and have just one afferent vessel, while malignant ones usually have several feeder vessels presenting with various wave shapes, simultaneous coexistence of low and high resistance flows, and a vascular network with disrupted architecture.

In particular, color Doppler is very helpful in rheumatology because it allows inactive pannus (almost avascular) to be discriminated from active (several blood spots inside); in this last case, the spectral analysis of the flow helps to distinguish the acute phase (with low resistance flows) from the chronic or quiescent one (where the resistances increase) [16-19].

Therefore, color Doppler is a technique that supplements the traditional B-mode imaging and can be very helpful when assessing muscular masses: it does not supply any further information about the nature of the lesion, but can provide important indications for a subsequent biopsy.

From a technical point of view, precise adjustment of Doppler parameters is highly recommended; the equipment must be set to assess low flows with low speed, applying low wall filters (WF) and pulse repetition frequency (PRF) between 700 Hz and 1 MHz. The gain is a separate consideration because it represents a parameter subjectively set by the operator. In rheumatology, the gain must be always set at the same level in order to follow up the modification of hyperemia and tissue perfusion inflammation during the progression of rheumatic pathology. With a thin layer of gel on the transducer, the operator can progressively increase the gain until some noise appears in the color box (1st phase) (Fig. 1.14); then the gain can be progressively decreased to reach a value just under the noise threshold (2nd phase) [20] (Fig. 1.15).

The recent introduction of intravenous contrast media for ultrasound has allowed even the smallest vessels – such as microcirculation capillaries – to be assessed, enhancing the incoming echoes.

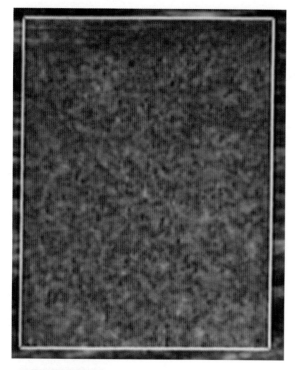

Fig. 1.14

Gain set (1st phase): the operator progressively increases the gain until some noise appears in the color box

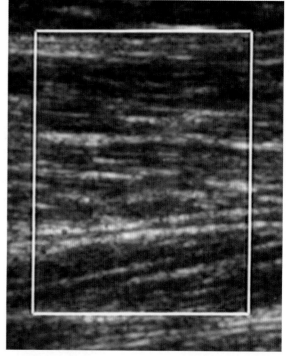

Fig. 1.15

Gain set (2nd phase): gain has been progressively decreased to reach the optimum value

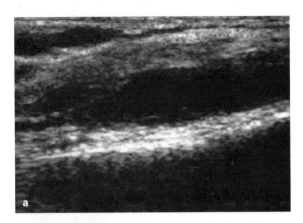 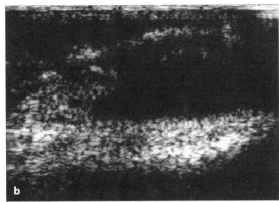

Fig. 1.16 a, b

Longitudinal US scan of suprapatellar recess in a rheumatoid patient. **a** B-mode US scan shows an effusion with a proliferative thickening of the synovial membrane. **b** After injection of intravenous sonographic contrast media, marked enhancement of the synovial proliferation is shown; this is directly related to neoangiogenic hyperemia

This has great relevance in rheumatology and, in particular, in the evaluation of the synovial membrane [4, 5, 21]. In fact, its vascularization consists of very small arterioles and venules and, when inflammatory pathology is in progress, they have very low flow that cannot be assessed using color Doppler alone.

1.5 Echo-contrast media

US contrast media consist of stabilized gas microbubbles which characteristically echo when hit by the US beam, and produce a very strong incoming echo. The most recent contrast media do not exit the vascular bed and therefore can help to assess very slow and low capillary flows. This feature allows the contrast media to reach tissues – like synovium – that are highly vascularized. It greatly increases the ability to assess the synovial membrane in inflammatory pathologies present-ing with angiogenesis and marked hyperemia [4, 5, 20] (Fig. 1.16 a, b).

Considering the high sensitivity of Doppler technique in rheumatology, the systematic use of contrast media is not necessary, but can be helpful during follow up. Recent studies have shown that it is possible to detect the effects of therapy on tissue perfusion after just a few weeks in patients affected by rheumatoid arthritis. In these situations, contrast media are a very precise means by which to highlight the amount of enhancement of the pannus before, during, and after treatment [5].

In addition, it is important to use wash-in and wash-out curves to assess perfusion in soft tissues [22]. Nevertheless, the use of the most recent generation of contrast media is strictly restricted by the availability of specific ultrasound equipment that are able to select a precise frequency band to assess the vascular enhancement caused by microbubbles. This is a further limitation to the diffusion of ultrasound contrast media.

References

1. Bude RO, Rubin JM (1996) Power Doppler sonography. Radiology 200:21
2. Breidahl WH, Newman JS, Toljanovic MS, Adler RS (1996) Power Doppler sonography in the assessment of musculoskeletal fluid collections. AJR Am J Roentgenol 166:1443-1446
3. Rubin JM (1994) Spectral Doppler US. RadioGraphics 14:139
4. Klauser A, Demharten J, De Marchi A et al (2005) Contrast enhanced gray-scale sonography in assessment of joint vascularity in rheumatoid arthritis: result from the IACUS study group. Eur Radiol 15:2404-2410
5. Salaffi F, Carotti M, Manganelli P et al (2004) Contrast-enhanced power Doppler sonography of knee synovitis in rheumatoid arthritis: assessment of therapeutic response. Clin Rheumatol 23:285-290

6. Lin EC, Middleton WD, Teefey SA (1999) Extended field of view sonography in musculoskeletal imaging. J ultrasound Med 18:147-152

7. Barberie JE, Wong AD, Cooperberg PL, Carson BW (1998) Extended field of view sonography in musculoskeletal disorders. AJR 171:751-757

8. Van Holsbeeck MT, Introcaso JH (2001) Musculoskeletal ultrasound, 2nd edition. Mosby, St. Louis

9. Teefey SA, Middleton WD, Yamaguchi K (1999) Shoulder sonography: state of the art. Radiol Clin North Am 37:767-785

10. Martinoli C, Bianchi S, Derchi LE (1999) Tendon and nerve sonography. Radiol Clin North Am 37:691-711

11. Silvestri E, Martinoli C, Derchi LE et al (1995) Echotexture of peripheral nerves: correlation between US and histologic findings and criteria to differentiate tendons. Radiology 197:291-296

12. Martinoli C, Derchi LE, Pastorino C et al (1993) Analysis of echotexture of tendons with US. Radiology 186:839-843

13. Silvestri E, La Paglia E, Avanzino C, Satragno L (2000) Hochauflosende Sonographie der Sehnen, Bander, peripheren Nerven und Muskeln: Eine neue Anatomie. Osterreichische Rontgen gesellschaft, pp 15-18

14. Rumack CM, Wilson SR, Charboneau JW, Johnson J (2004) Diagnostic Ultrasound, 3rd edition. Mosby, St. Louis

15. Kremkau FW (1990) Chapter 4: Doppler effect. In: Doppler ultrasound: principles and instruments. W.B. Saunders

16. Newman JS, Adler RS, Bude RO, Rubin JM (1994) Detection of soft-tissue hyperemia: value of power Doppler sonography. AJR 163:385-389

17. Kane D, Grassi W, Sturrock R, Balint PV (2004) Musculoskeletal ultrasound–a state of the art review in rheumatology. Part 2: Clinical indications for musculoskeletal ultrasound in rheumatology. Rheumatology 43:829-838

18. Kane DJ, Balint PV, Sturrock R, Grassi W (2004) Musculoskeletal ultrasound - a state of the art review in rheumatology. Part 1: Current controversies and issues in the development of musculoskeletal ultrasound in rheumatology. Rheumatology 43:823-828

19. Wakefield RJ, Brown AK, Emery P (2003) Power Doppler sonography: improving disease activity assessment in inflammatory joint disease. Arthritis Rheum 48:285-289

20. Rubin JM, Bude RO, Carson PL et al (1994) Power Doppler US: a potentially useful alternative to mean frequency- based color Doppler US. Radiology 190:853

21. Carotti M, Salaffi F, De Bernardis S, Argalia G (2000) Color Power Doppler e mezzi di contrasto nello studio della membrana sinoviale del ginocchio nell'artrite reumatoide. Progressi in Reumatologia 6(vol I):63-75

22. Eggermont AM (2005) Evolving imaging technology: contrast enhanced Doppler ultrasound is early and rapid predictor of tumors response. Ann Oncol 16:1054-1060

Examination technique and procedure

2.1 Thoracic and abdominal wall

THORACIC WALL

Longitudinal view
Sternocostal joint

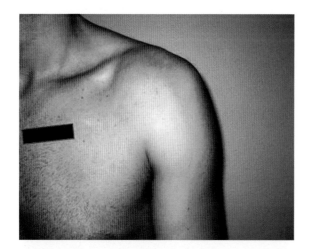

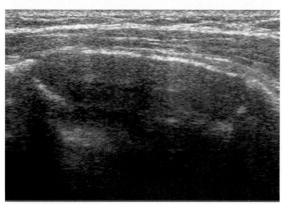

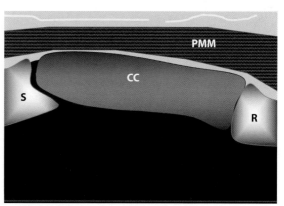

Fig. 2.1

Sternocostal longitudinal view. *R* = rib; *S* = sternum; *CC* = costal cartilage; *PMM* = pectoralis major muscle

THORACIC WALL
Longitudinal view
Sternoclavicular joint

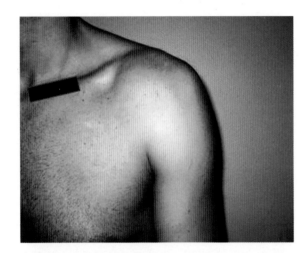

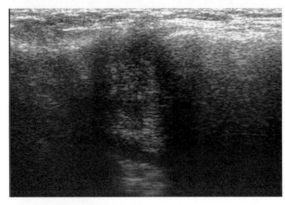
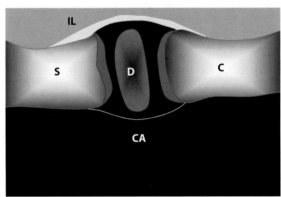

Fig. 2.2

Sternoclavicular longitudinal view. C = clavicle; S = sternum; D = articular disk; CA = capsule; IL = interclavicular ligament

ABDOMINAL WALL
Axial view
Rectus abdomini muscles

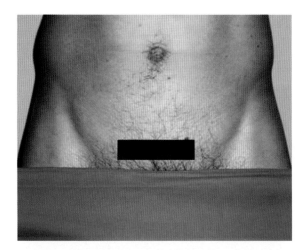

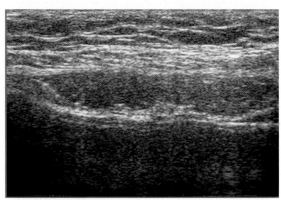

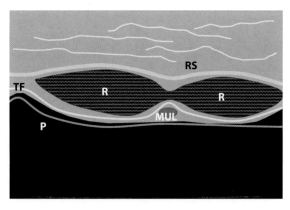

Fig. 2.3

Axial view of rectus abdomini muscles. *R* = rectus abdominis muscle; *TF* = transversalis fascia; *RS* = rectus sheath; *MUL* = medial umbilical ligament-obliterated urachus; *P* = peritoneum

ABDOMINAL WALL
Longitudinal view
Rectus abdominis muscle

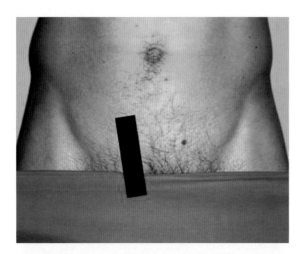

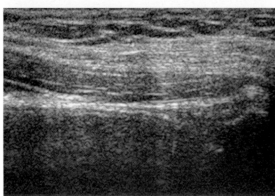

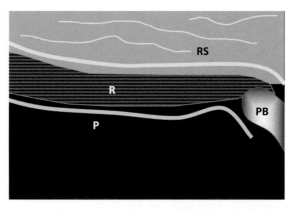

Fig. 2.4

Longitudinal view of rectus abdominis muscle. *R* = rectus abdominis muscle; *RS* = rectus sheath; *PB* = pubic bone; *P* = peritoneum

2.2 Upper extremity

SHOULDER
Short axis view
Subscapularis tendon

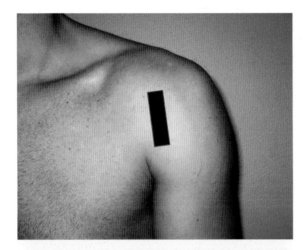

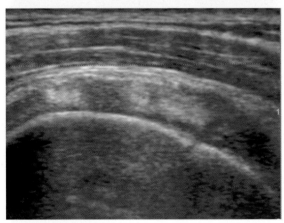
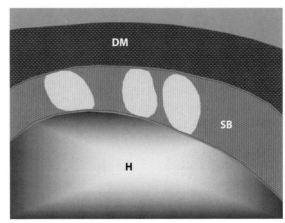

Fig. 2.5

Short axis view of subscapularis tendon. *H* = humerus; *SB* = subscapularis tendon; *DM* = deltoid muscle

tendon has 3 bundles

SHOULDER

Long axis view
Subscapularis tendon

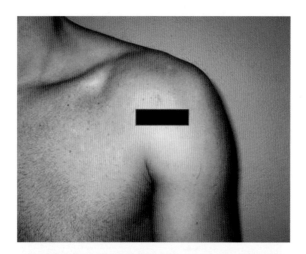

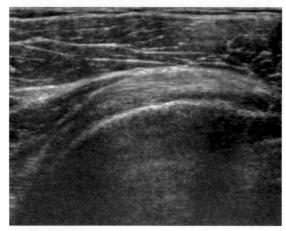 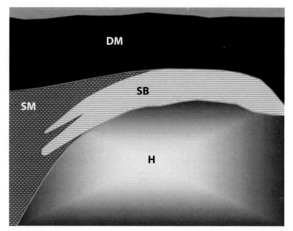

Fig. 2.6

Long axis scan of subscapularis tendon. *H* = humerus; *SB* = subscapularis tendon; *SM* = subscapularis muscle; *DM* = deltoid muscle

SHOULDER
Long axis view
Supraspinatus tendon

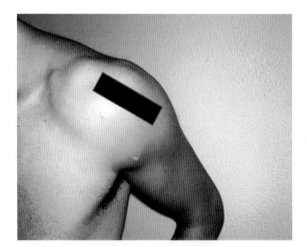

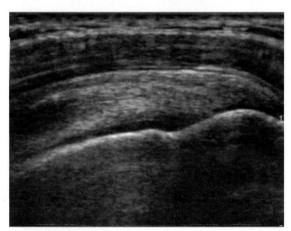
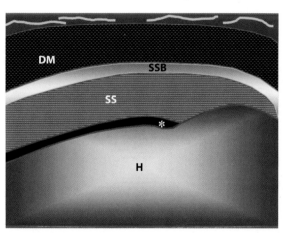

Fig. 2.7

Long axis view of supraspinatus tendon. *H* = humerus; *SS* = supraspinatus tendon; *SSB* = subacromial subdeltoid bursa; *DM* = deltoid muscle; * = articular cartilage

SHOULDER
Axial view
Rotator interval

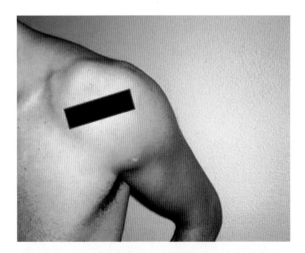

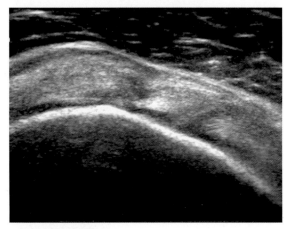

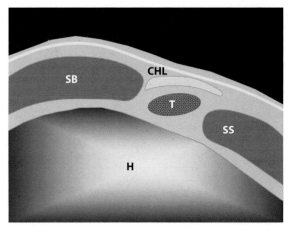

Fig. 2.8

Axial view of rotator interval. *H* = humerus; *SS* = supraspinatus tendon short axis; *SB* = subscapularis tendon short axis; *T* = long head biceps tendon; *CHL* = coraco humeral ligament

SHOULDER
Long axis view
Infraspinatus tendon

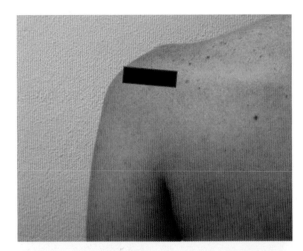

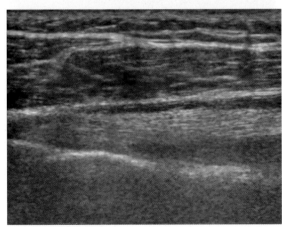
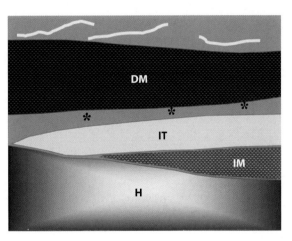

Fig. 2.9

Long axis view of infraspinatus tendon. *H* = humerus; *IT* = infraspinatus tendon; *IM* = infraspinatus muscle; * = subacromial sub-deltoid bursa; *DM* = deltoid muscle

SHOULDER

Short axis view
Infraspinatus and teres minor tendons

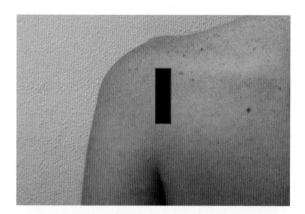

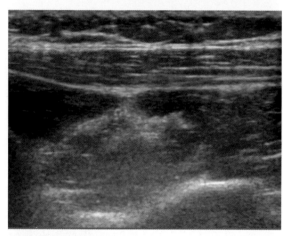 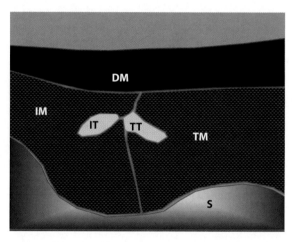

Fig. 2.10

Short axis view of infraspinatus and teres minor tendons. *S* = scapula; *IT* = infraspinatus tendon; *IM* = infraspinatus muscle; *TT* = teres minor tendon; *TM* = teres minor muscle; *DM* = deltoid muscle

SHOULDER
Short axis view
Long head of biceps tendon

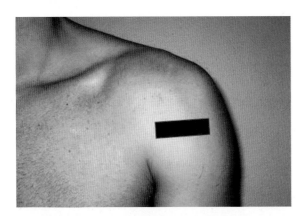

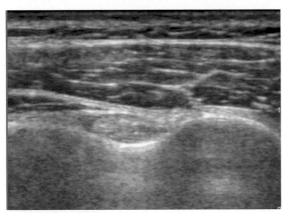
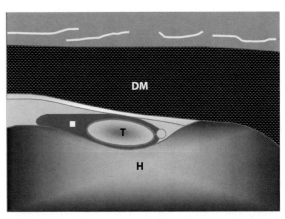

Fig. 2.11 a

Axial view of long head of biceps tendon. *H* = humerus; *T* = long head of the biceps tendon; □ = tendon sheath; *DM* = deltoid muscle

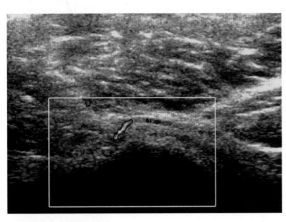
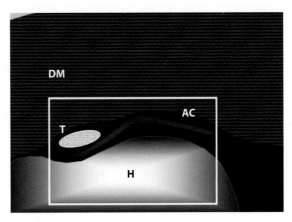

Fig. 2.11 b

Anterior circumflex humeral artery (Color Doppler). *H* = humerus; *AC* = anterior circumflex humeral artery; *T* = long head of biceps tendon; *DM* = deltoid muscle

SHOULDER

Long axis view
Long head of biceps tendon

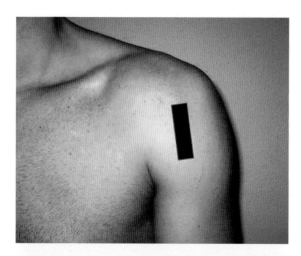

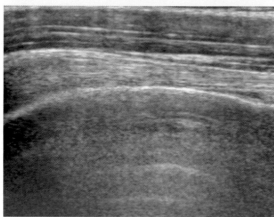

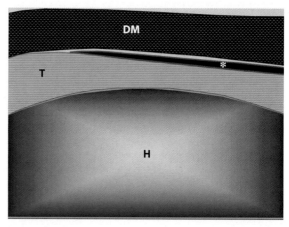

Fig. 2.12

Longitudinal view of long head of biceps tendon. *H* = humerus; *T* = long head of the biceps tendon; * = tendon sheath; *DM* = deltoid muscle

SHOULDER
Axial view
Pectoralis major tendon

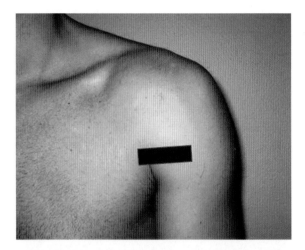

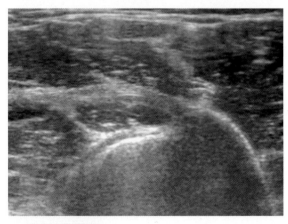

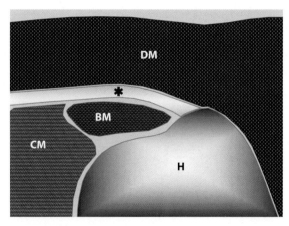

Fig. 2.13

Axial view of pectoralis major tendon. *H* = humerus; *BM* = short head of biceps muscle; *CM* = coracobrachialis muscle; * = pectoralis major tendon; *DM* = deltoid muscle

SHOULDER
Longitudinal view
Coraco-acromial ligament

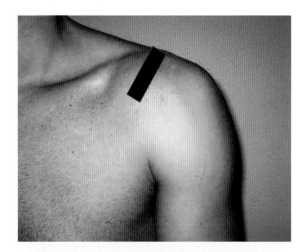

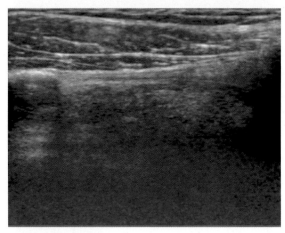
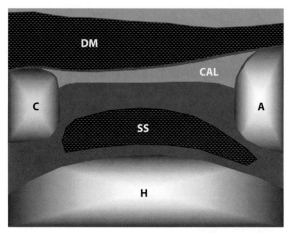

Fig. 2.14

Longitudinal view of coraco-acromial ligament. *H* = humerus; *C* = coracoid process; *A* = acromion; *SS* = supraspinatus tendon; *CAL* = coraco-acromial ligament; *DM* = deltoid muscle

SHOULDER
Longitudinal view
Acromio-clavicular joint

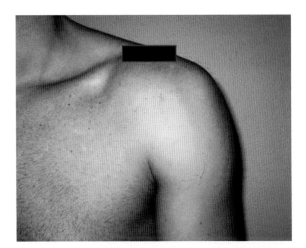

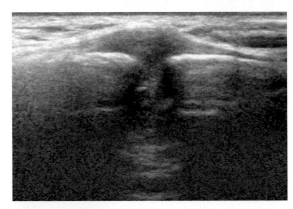 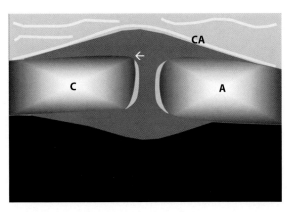

Fig. 2.15

Longitudinal view of acromio-clavicular joint. *C* = clavicle; *A* = acromion; *CA* = capsule; ← = synovial space

SHOULDER
Longitudinal view
Axillary recess

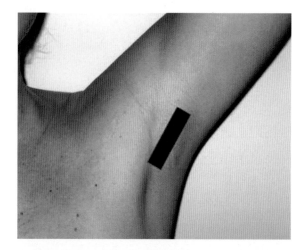

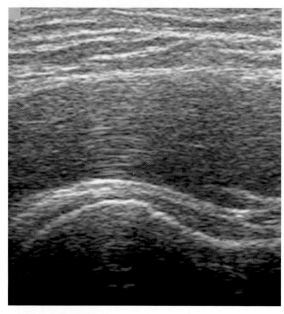

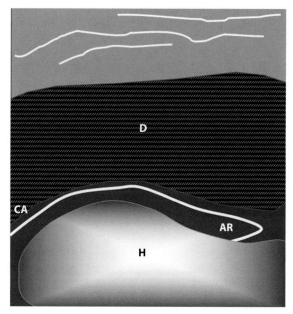

Fig. 2.16

Longitudinal view of axillary recess. *H* = humerus; *AR* = axillary recess; *CA* = capsule; *D* = latissimus dorsi muscle

ELBOW LATERAL
Long axis view
Common extensor tendon insertion

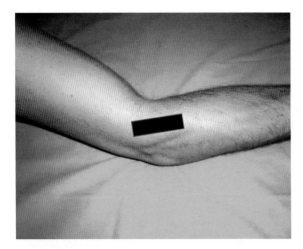

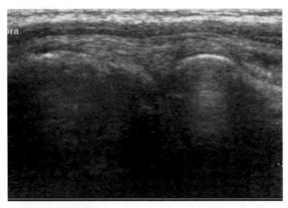

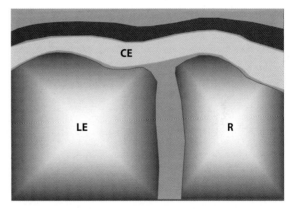

Fig. 2.17

Long axis view of common extensor tendon insertion. *CE* = extensor tendons insertion; *LE* = lateral epycondyle; *R* = radial head

ELBOW MEDIAL
Long axis view
Common flexor tendon insertion

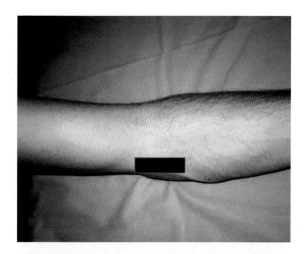

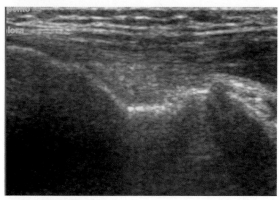

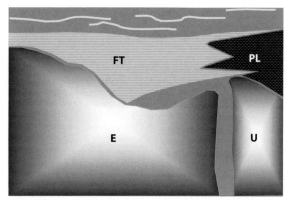

Fig. 2.18

Long axis view of the common flexor tendon insertion. *E* = medial epycondyle; *U* = ulna; *FT* = common flexor tendon; *PL* = pal-maris longus muscle

ELBOW ANTERIOR
Long axis view
Distal biceps tendon

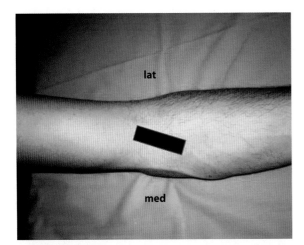

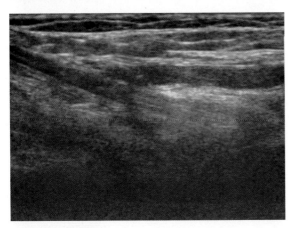

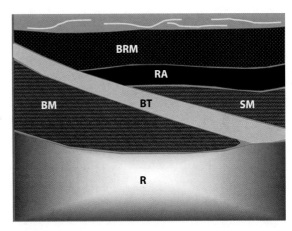

Fig. 2.19

Long axis view of distal biceps tendon. *R* = radium; *BT* = distal biceps tendon; *BM* = brachial muscle; *SM* = supinator muscle; *RA* = radial artery; *BRM* = brachioradialis muscle; *med* = medial (ulnar) aspect; *lat* = lateral (radial) aspect

ELBOW POSTERIOR
Long axis view
Triceps tendon

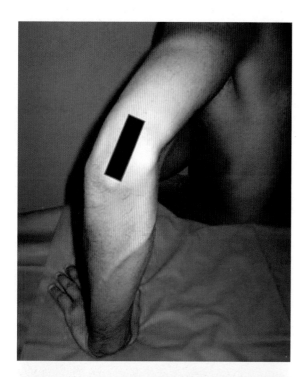

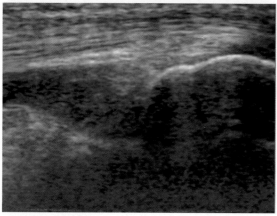 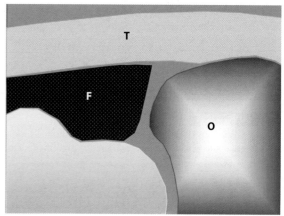

Fig. 2.20

Long axis view of the triceps tendon. *O* = olecranon; *F* = fat pad; *T* = triceps tendon

ELBOW ANTERIOR
Axial view
Median nerve

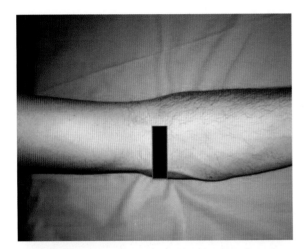

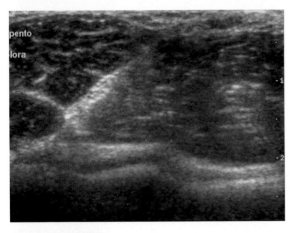

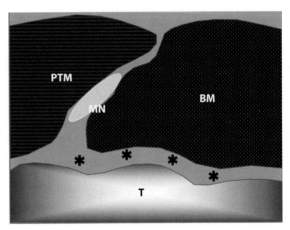

Fig. 2.21

Short axis view of medial nerve. *T* = humeral trochlea; *MN* = median nerve; *BM* = brachial muscle; *PTM* = pronator teres muscle; * = articular cartilage

ELBOW ANTERIOR
Long axis view
Median nerve

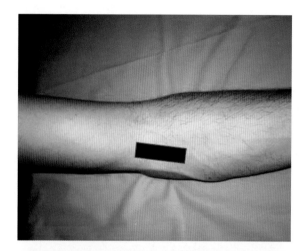

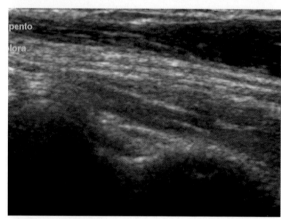

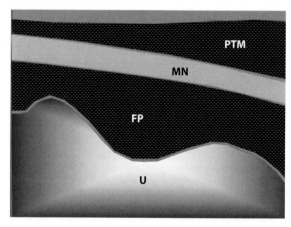

Fig. 2.22

Long axis view of median nerve. *U* = ulna; *FP* = flexor digitorum profundus muscle; *MN* = median nerve; *PTM* = pronator teres muscle

ELBOW ANTERIOR
Short axis view
Radial nerve

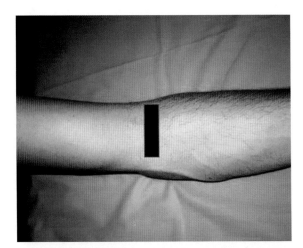

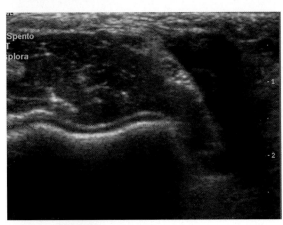

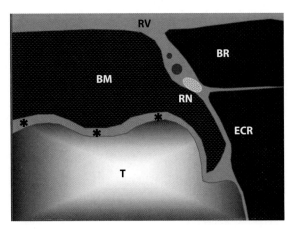

Fig. 2.23

Short axis view of radial nerve. *T* = humeral trochlea; *BM* = brachialis muscle; *BR* = brachioradialis muscle; *ECR* = extensor carpi radialis longus muscle; *RV* = radial vessels; *RN* = radial nerve; * = articular cartilage

ELBOW ANTERIOR
Short axis view (Doppler)

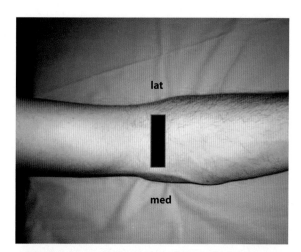

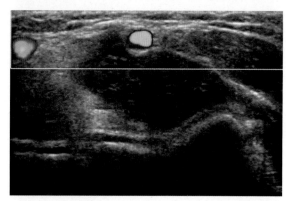
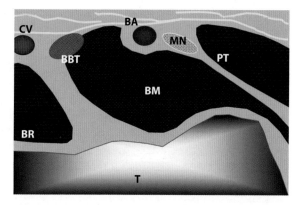

Fig. 2.24

Color Doppler of the anterior aspect of the elbow (axial view). *T* = humeral trochlea; *BR* = brachioradialis muscle; *PT* = pronator teres muscle; *BM* = brachialis muscle; *BA* = brachial artery; *CV* = cephalic vein; *BBT* = brachial biceps tendon; *MN* = median nerve; *med* = medial (ulnar) aspect; *lat* = lateral (radial) aspect

ELBOW ANTERIOR
Long axis view
Radial nerve

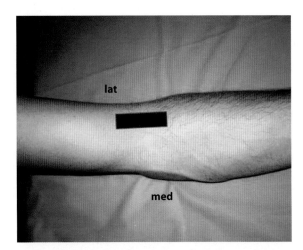

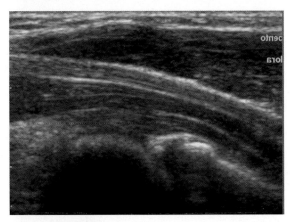

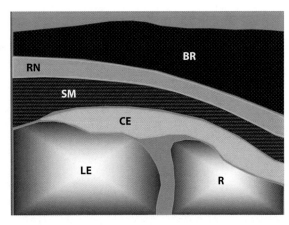

Fig. 2.25

Long axis view of radial nerve. *LE* = lateral epicondyle; *R* = radial head; *CE* = common extensor tendon; *SM* = supinator muscle; *BR* = brachioradialis muscle; *RN* = radial nerve; *med* = medial (ulnar) aspect; *lat* = lateral (radial) aspect

ELBOW ANTERIOR
Short axis view
Radial nerve (arcade of Frohse)

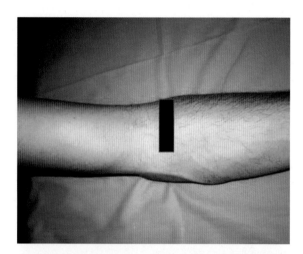

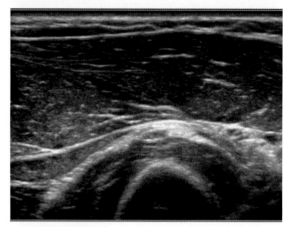
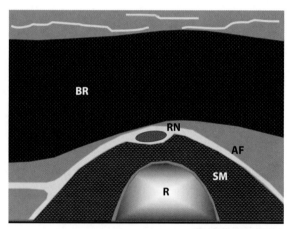

Fig. 2.26

Axial view of radial nerve at the level of the arcade of Frohse. *R* = radius; *BR* = brachioradialis muscle; *RN* = radial nerve; *AF* = arcade of Frohse; *SM* = supinator muscle

ELBOW POSTERIOR
Short axis view
Ulnar nerve

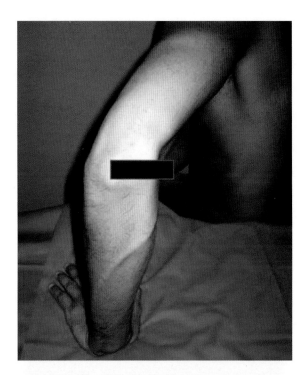

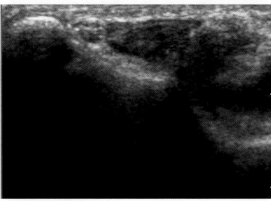

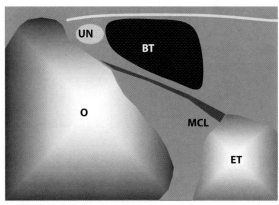

Fig. 2.27

Short axis view of the ulnar nerve at the groove formed by the medial epicondyle and olecranon. *O* =olecranon; *ME* = medial epicondyle; *BT* = Brachialis triceps muscle (medial belly); *MCL* = medial collateral ligament; *UN* = ulnar nerve

ELBOW POSTERIOR
Short axis view
Ulnare nerve (cubital tunnel)

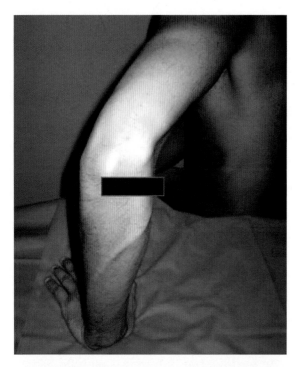

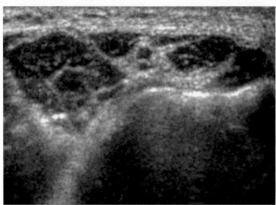

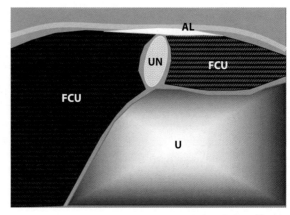

Fig. 2.28

Axial view of the cubital tunnel. *U* = ulna; *UN* = ulnar nerve; *FCU* = flexor carpi ulnaris muscle; *AL* = arcuate ligament

ELBOW POSTERIOR
Long axis view
Ulnar nerve

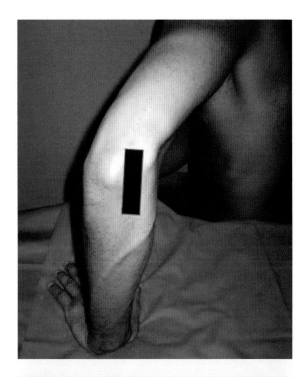

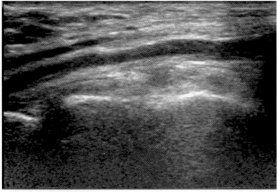

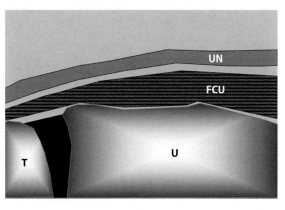

Fig. 2.29

Long axis view of the ulnar nerve. *U* = ulna; *T* = humeral trochlea; *UN* = ulnar nerve; *FCU* = flexor carpi ulnaris muscle

ELBOW ANTERIOR
Longitudinal view (radial side)

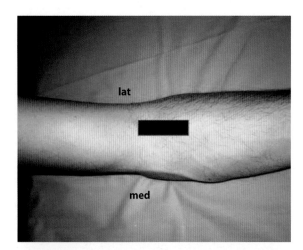

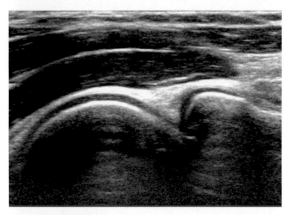
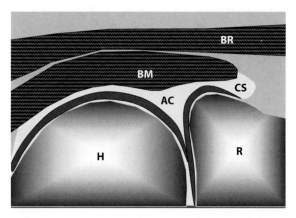

Fig. 2.30

Longitudinal view of the anterior aspect of the elbow (radial side). *H* = humerus; *R* = radial head, *AC* = articular cartilage; *CS* = capsule and humeroradial synovial space; *BM* = brachialis muscle; *BR* = brachioradialis muscle; *med* = medial (ulnar) aspect; *lat* = lateral (radial) aspect

ELBOW ANTERIOR
Longitudinal view (ulnar side)

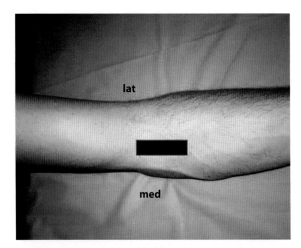

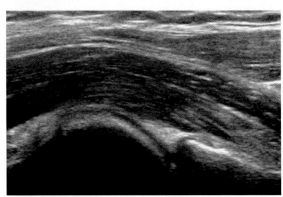

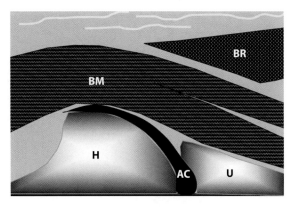

Fig. 2.31

Longitudinal view of the anterior aspect of the elbow (ulnar side). *H* = humerus; *U* = ulna; *AC* = articular cartilage; *BM* = brachialis muscle; *BR* = brachioradialis muscle ; *med* = medial (ulnar) aspect; *lat* = lateral (radial) aspect

WRIST

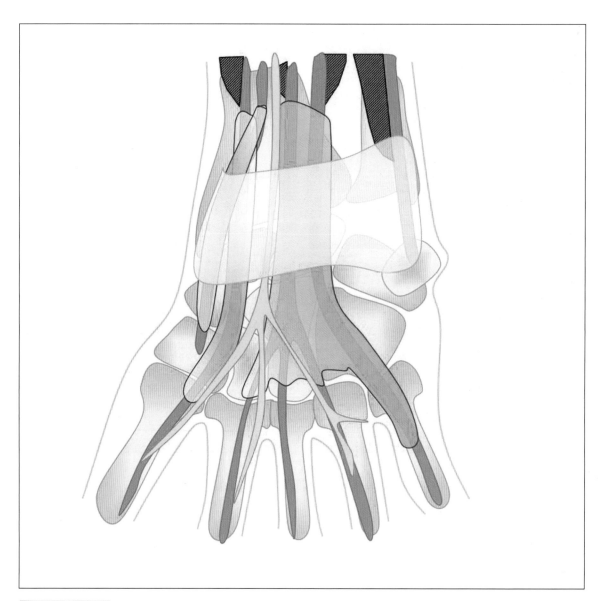

Fig. 2.32

Anatomic diagram of the wrist

WRIST VOLAR
Axial view
Carpal tunnel

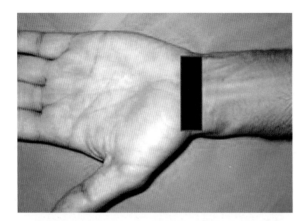

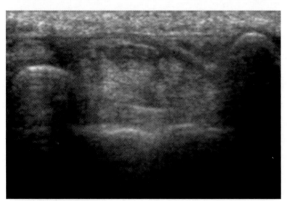
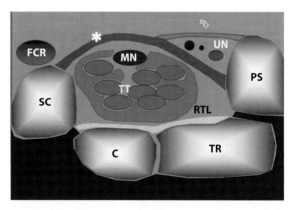

Fig. 2.33

Proximal axial view of the carpal tunnel. *SC* = scaphoid; *C* = capitate; *TR* = triquetrum; *PS* = pisiform; * =flexor retinaculum (transverse ligament); *TT* = profundus and superficialis flexor tendons ; *MN* = median nerve ; *UN* = ulnar nerve (⇗ Guyon tunnel); *RTL* = radio-triquetral palmar ligament; *FCR* = flexor carpi radialis tendon

WRIST VOLAR
Axial view
Carpal tunnel

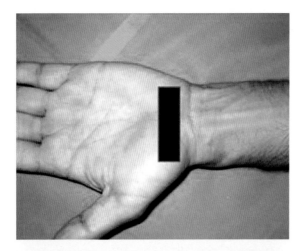

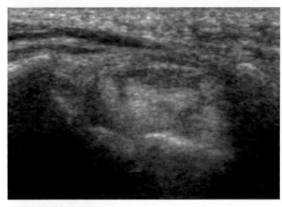

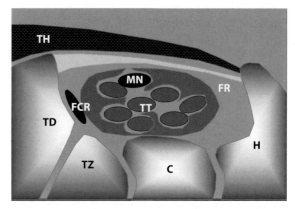

Fig. 2.34

Distal axial view of the carpal tunnel. *TD* = trapezoid; *TZ* = trapezium; *C* = capitate; *H* = hamate; *FR* = flexor retinaculum; *TT* = profundus and superficialis flexor tendons; *MN* = median nerve; *FCR* = flexor carpi radialis tendon; *TH* = thenar eminence muscles

WRIST VOLAR
Longitudinal view
Flexor tendons

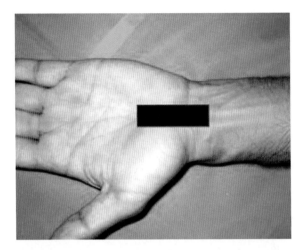

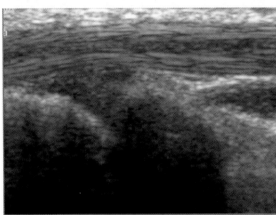

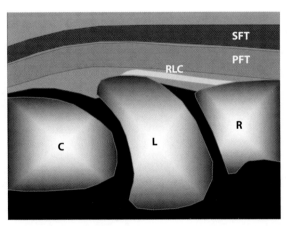

Fig. 2.35

Long axis view of flexor tendons. *R* = radius; *L* = lunate; *C* = capitate; *PFT* = profundus flexor tendons; *SFT* = superficialis flexor tendons; *RLC* = radio-luno-capitate ligament

WRIST VOLAR
Longitudinal view
Carpal tunnel (median nerve)

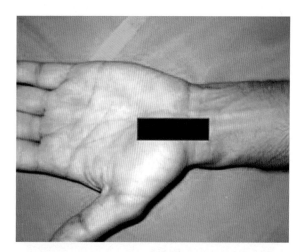

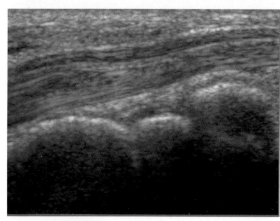

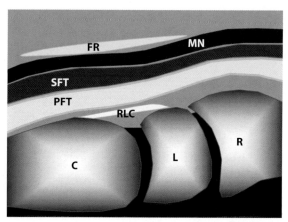

Fig. 2.36

Carpal tunnel: long axis view of the median nerve. *R* = radius; *L* = lunate; *C* = capitate; *PFT* = profundus flexor tendons; *SFT* = superficialis flexor tendons; *RLC* = radio-luno-capitate ligament; *MN* = median nerve; *FR* = flexor retinaculum

WRIST DORSAL
Dorsal axial view
Extensor tendons

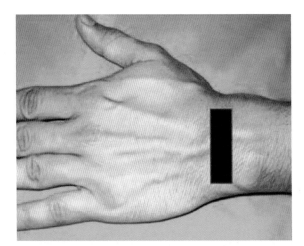

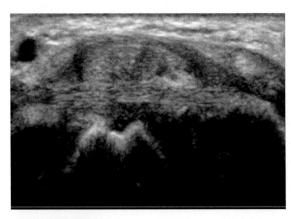

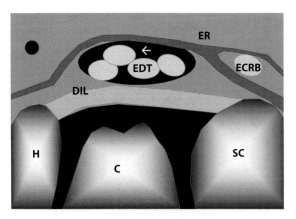

Fig. 2.37

Extensor tendons (dorsal axial view). *H* = hamate; *C* = capitate; *SC* = scaphoid; *DIL* = dorsal intercarpal ligament; *EDT* = extensor digitorum tendons; *ECRB* = extensor carpi radialis brevis; *ER* = extensor retinaculum; ← = common tendon sheath of the extensor tendons

WRIST LATERAL
Axial view
First dorsal compartment

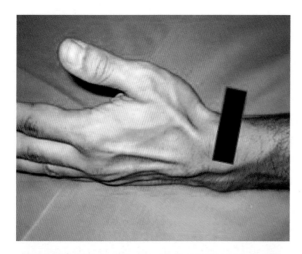

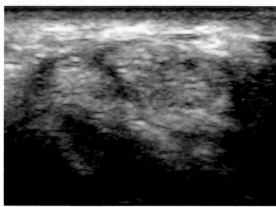

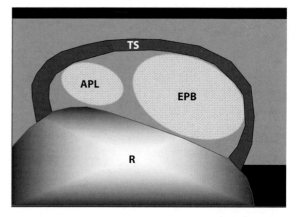

Fig. 2.38

Axial view of first dorsal compartment. *R* = radium; *APL* = abductor pollicis longus tendon; *EPB* = extensor pollicis brevis; *TS* = tendon sheath

WRIST MEDIAL
Longitudinal view
Triangular fibrocartilage

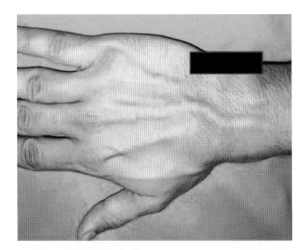

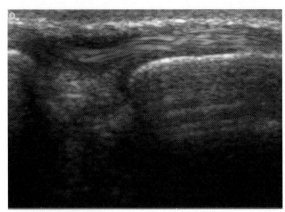
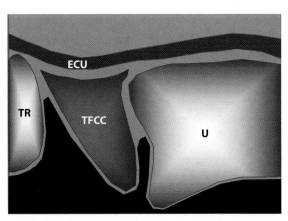

Fig. 2.39

Longitudinal view of triangular fibrocartilage. *U* = ulna; *TR* = triquetrum; *TFCC* = triangular fibrocartilage complex; *ECU* = extensor carpi ulnaris tendon

HAND PALMAR
Axial view
Flexor tendons

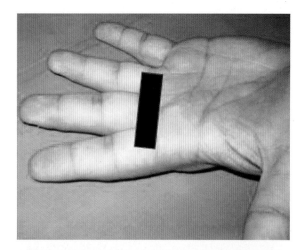

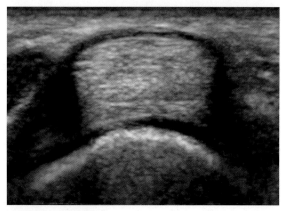 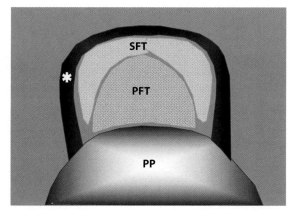

Fig. 2.40

Axial view of the finger, volar aspect. *PP* = proximal phalanx; *PFT* = profundus flexor tendon; *SFT* = superficialis flexor tendon (cranially to the division in the two lateral branches); * = flexor tendon pulley (A1)

HAND PALMAR
Longitudinal view
Flexor tendons

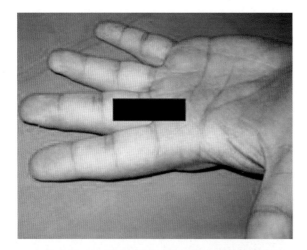

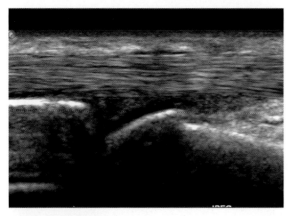
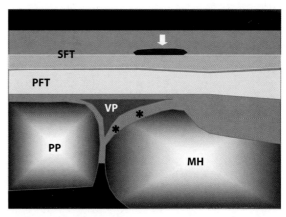

Fig. 2.41

Longitudinal view of the finger, volar aspect. *PP* = proximal phalanx; *MH* = metacarpal head; *VP* = volar plate; * = articular cartilage; *PFT* = profundus flexor tendon; *SFT* = superficialis flexor tendon; ⇩ = flexor tendon pulley (A1)

2.3 Lower extremity

HIP ANTERIOR

Longitudinal view
Coxofemoral joint

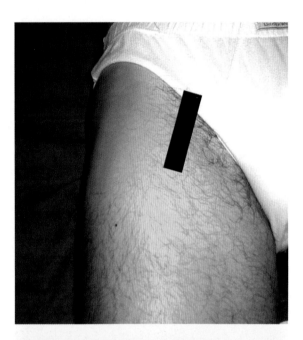

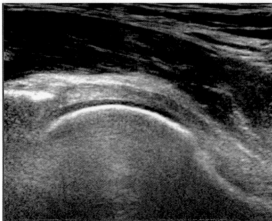

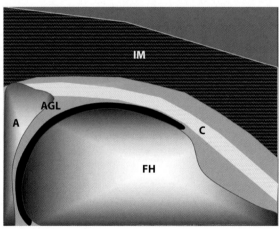

Fig. 2.42

Anterior view of coxofemoral joint. *IM* = ileopsoas muscle; *A* = acetabulum; *AGL* = anterior glenoid labrum of the acetabulum; *FH* = femoral head; *C* = capsule and anterior joint recess

HIP MEDIAL

Longitudinal view
Adductor muscles insertion

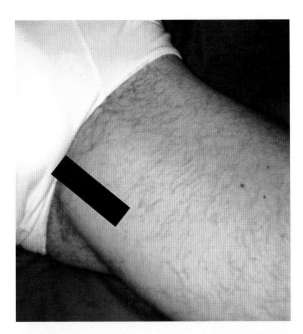

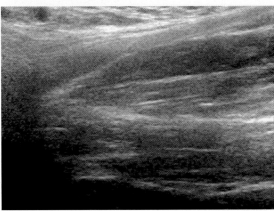
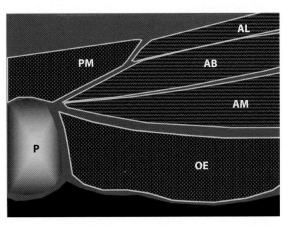

Fig. 2.43

Longitudinal view of adductor muscles. *P* = pubis; *OE* = obturator externus; *AM* = adductor magnus muscle; *AB* = adductor brevis muscle; *AL* = adductor longus muscle; *PM* = pectineus muscle

HIP POSTERIOR

Longitudinal view
Gluteus muscles

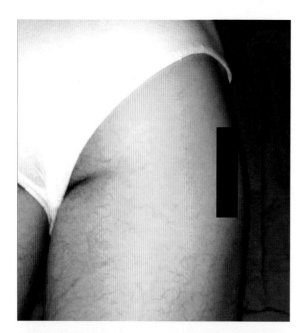

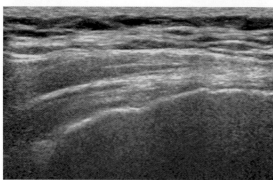

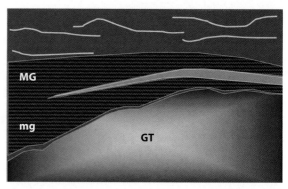

Fig. 2.44

Longitudinal view of gluteus minimus and gluteus medius at the greater trochanter. *GT* = greater trochanter; *mg* = gluteus minimus muscle and tendons; *MG* = gluteus medius muscle and tendons

HIP MEDIAL
Longitudinal view
Ileopsoas muscle insertion

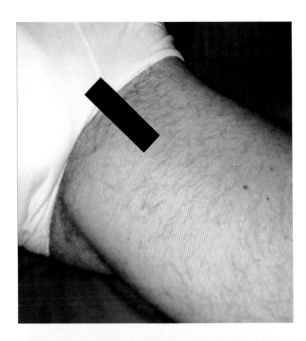

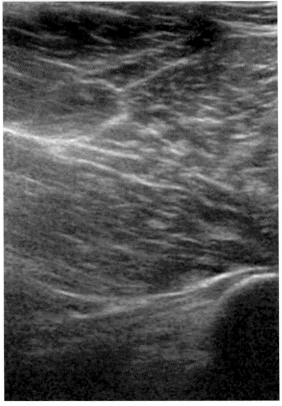

Fig. 2.45

Longitudinal view of ileopsoas muscle insertion at the lesser trochanter. *LT* = lesser trochanter; *IP* = ileopsoas muscle and tendon; *PM* = pectineus muscle; *AM* = adductor magnus

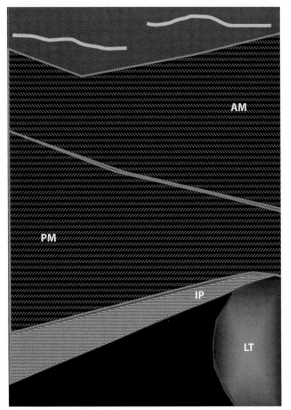

HIP POSTERIOR
Longitudinal view
Hamstrings

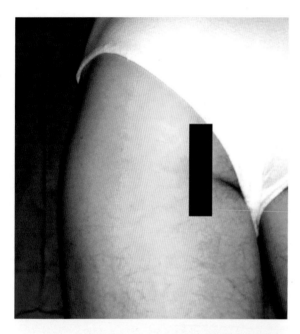

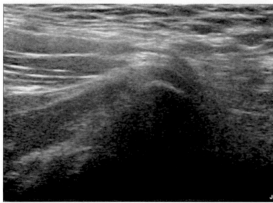

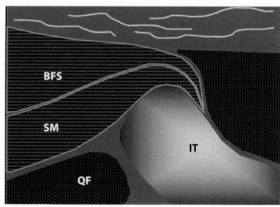

Fig. 2.46

Longitudinal view of extensor tendons (hamstrings) at the ischial tuberosity. *IT* = ischial tuberosity; *QF* = quadratus femoris; *SM* = semimembranosus muscle and tendon; *BFS* = biceps femoris and semitendinosus muscles and tendons

HIP POSTERIOR
Short axis view
Sciatic nerve

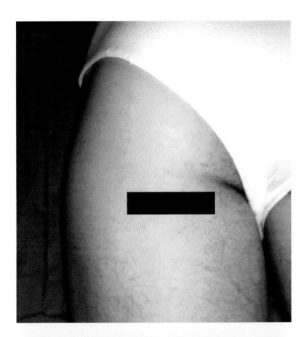

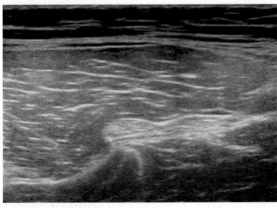

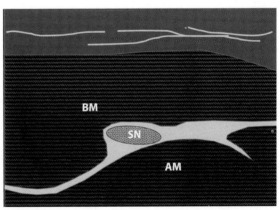

Fig. 2.47

Short axis view of sciatic nerve. *SN* = sciatic nerve; *AM* = adductor magnus muscle; *BM* = long head of biceps muscle

HIP POSTERIOR
Long axis view
Sciatic nerve

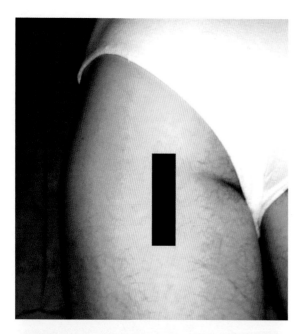

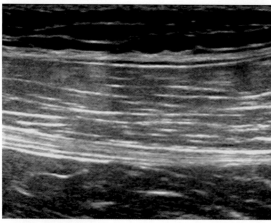

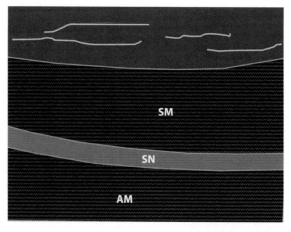

Fig. 2.48

Long axis view of the sciatic nerve. *SN* = sciatic nerve; *SM* = semitendinosus muscle; *AM* = adductor magnus muscle

HIP ANTERIOR
Longitudinal view
Femoral vessels (Doppler)

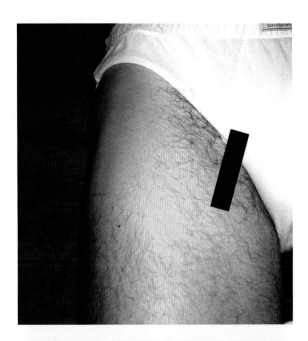

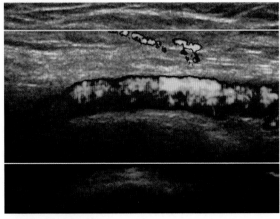

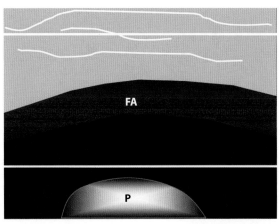

Fig. 2.49

Longitudinal view of femoral vessels. *P* = pubis; *FA* = femoral artery

HIP ANTERIOR
Axial view
Femoral vessels (Doppler)

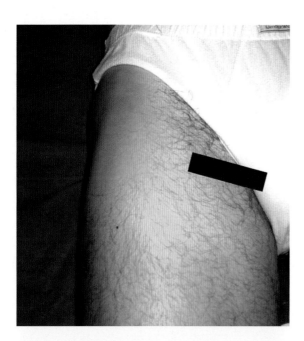

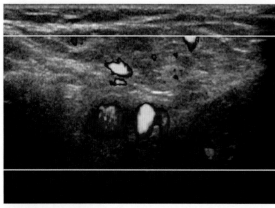

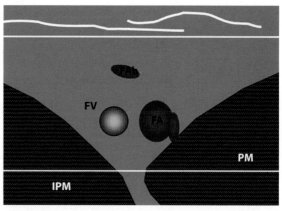

Fig. 2.50

Axial view of femoral vessels. *FV* = femoral vein; *FA* = femoral artery at the division of the deep femoral artery; *FAb* = femoral artery branch (medial cinconflex femoral artery); *PM* = pectineus muscle; *IPM* = ileopsoas muscle

HIP ANTERIOR
Longitudinal view
Antero-inferior iliac spine

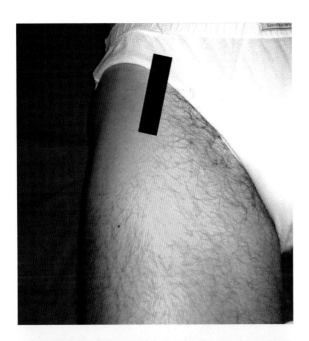

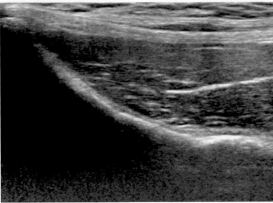

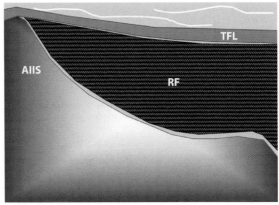

Fig. 2.51

Longitudinal view of antero-inferior iliac spine. *AIIS* = antero-inferior iliac spine; *TFL* = tensor fasciae latae muscle; *RF* = rectus femoris muscle

KNEE POSTERIOR
Longitudinal view
Medial meniscus

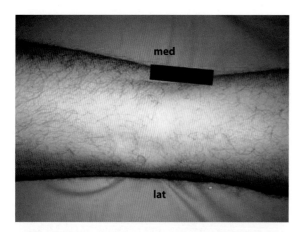

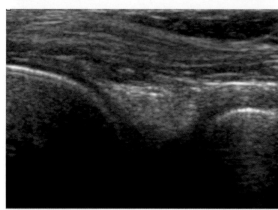

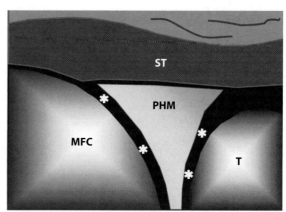

Fig. 2.52

Longitudinal view of the posterior horn of the medial meniscus. *T* = tibia; *PHM* = posterior horn of the medial meniscus; *MFC* = medial femoral condyle; *ST* = semimembranosus tendon; * = articular cartilage

KNEE MEDIAL

Longitudinal view
Medial collateral ligament

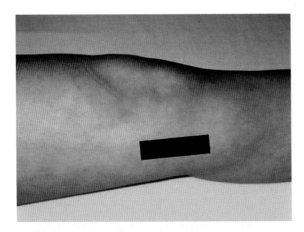

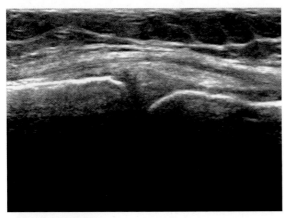

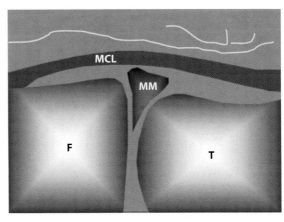

Fig. 2.53

Longitudinal view of the medial collateral ligament. *F* = femoral condyle; *T* = tibia; *MM* = medial meniscus; *MCL* = medial collateral ligament

KNEE POSTERIOR
Longitudinal view
Lateral meniscus

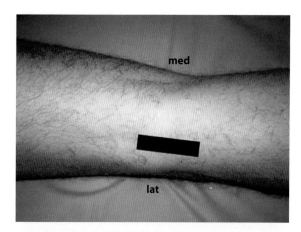

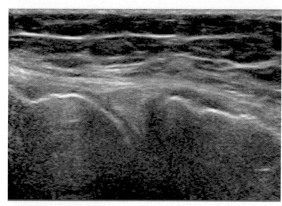

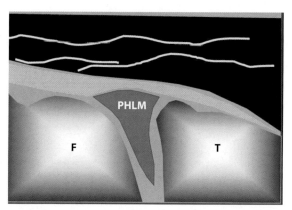

Fig. 2.54

Longitudinal view of lateral meniscus. *PHLM* = posterior horn of lateral meniscus; *F* = lateral femoral condyle; *T* = tibia

KNEE LATERAL
Longitudinal view
Lateral collateral ligament

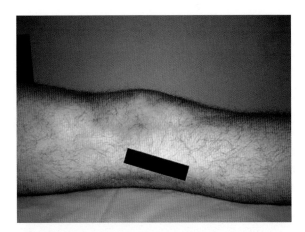

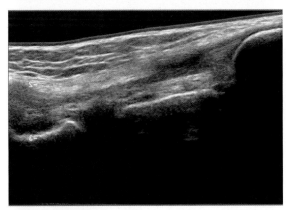
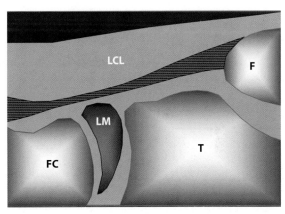

Fig. 2.55

Longitudinal view of the lateral collateral ligament. *LCL* = lateral collateral ligament; *LM* = lateral meniscus; *FC* = lateral femoral condyle; *F* = fibula; *T* = tibia

KNEE ANTERIOR
Short axis view
Patellar tendon

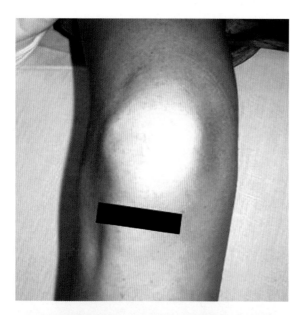

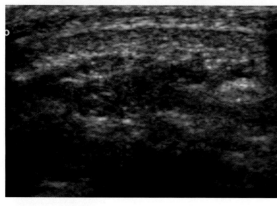

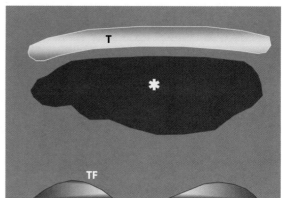

Fig. 2.56

Short axis view of the patellar tendon. *T* = patellar tendon; * = Hoffa's pad; *TF* = femoral trochlea

KNEE ANTERIOR
Long axis view
Patellar tendon

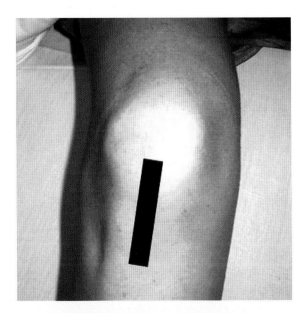

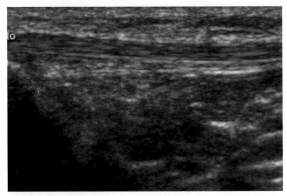

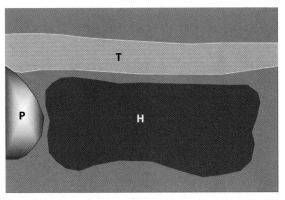

Fig. 2.57

Long axis view of the patellar tendon. *T* = patellar tendon; *H* = Hoffa's pad; *P* = patella

KNEE ANTERIOR
Longitudinal view
Quadriceps tendon and suprapatellar recess

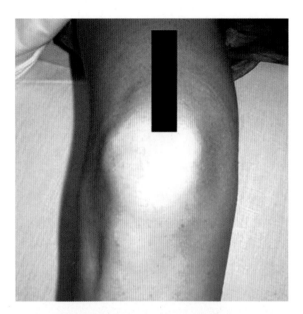

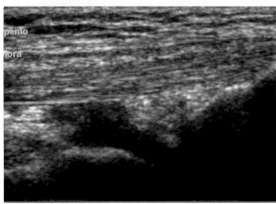

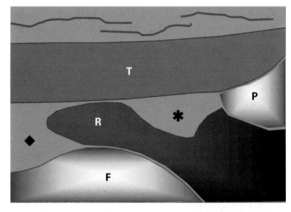

Fig. 2.58

Longitudinal view of quadriceps tendon and suprapatellar recess. *T* = quadriceps tendon; *P* = patella; *R* = suprapatellar recess; * = suprapatellar fat pad; ◆ = pre femoral fat pad; *F* = femur

KNEE LATERAL
Short axis view
Popliteus tendon

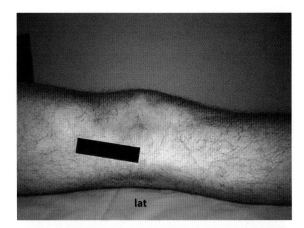

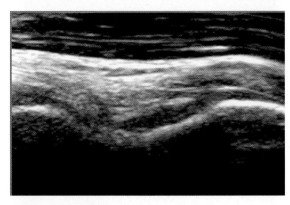

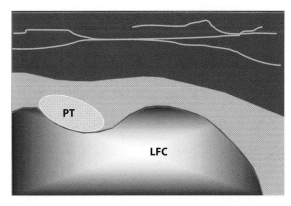

Fig. 2.59

Short axis view of the popliteus tendon (longitudinal scan of the lateral aspect of the knee). *PT* = popliteus tendon; *LFC* = lateral femoral condyle

KNEE LATERAL
Long axis view
Ileotibial band

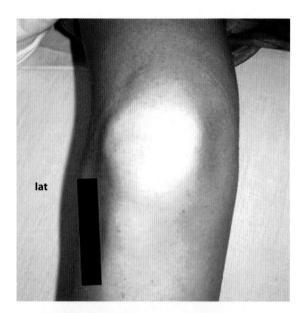

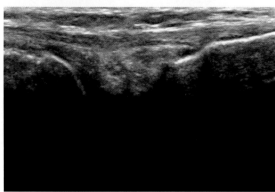

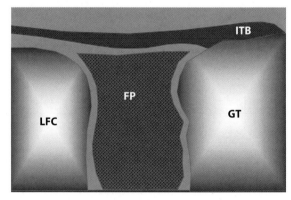

Fig. 2.60

Long axis view of the ileotibial band. *ITB* = ileotibial band; *GT* = Gerdy's tubercle (ileotibial band insertion); *FP* = fat pad; *LFC* = lateral femoral condyle

KNEE MEDIAL
Longitudinal view
Pes anserina

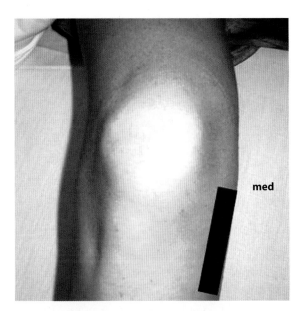

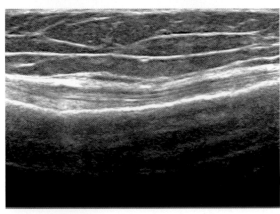
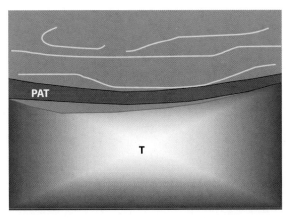

Fig. 2.61

Longitudinal view of pes anserina. *T* = tibia; *PAT* = pes anserina tendons, (gracilis, sartorius and semitendinosus); *med* = medial aspect

KNEE ANTERIOR
Axial view
Femoral trochlea

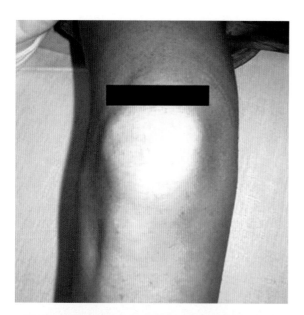

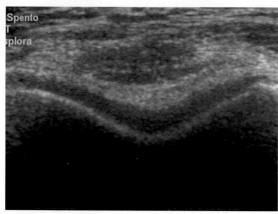

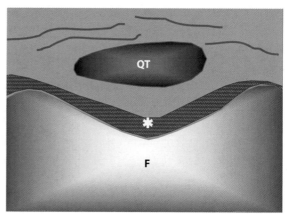

Fig. 2.62

Femoral trochlea (axial scan). *F* = femoral trochlea; * = articular cartilage; *QT* = quadriceps tendon

KNEE POSTERIOR
Long axis view
Common peroneal nerve

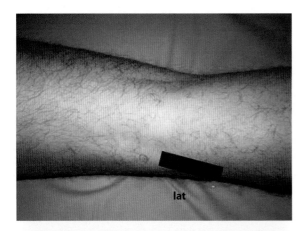

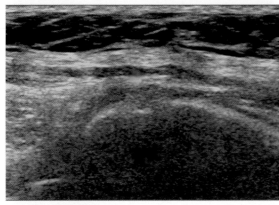
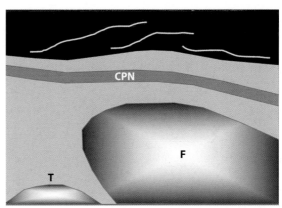

Fig. 2.63

Long axis view of the common peroneal nerve. *CPN* = common peroneal nerve; *T* = tibia; *F* = fibula; *lat* = lateral aspect

KNEE POSTERIOR
Short axis view
Common peroneal nerve

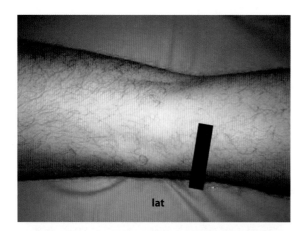

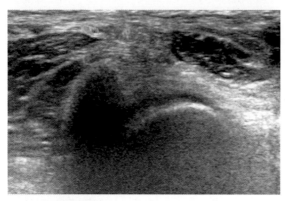
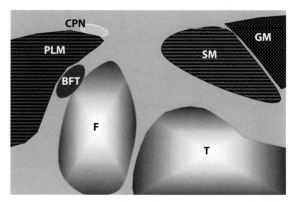

Fig. 2.64

Short axis view of the common peroneal nerve. *CPN* = common peroneal nerve; *PLM* = peroneus longus muscle; *BFT* = biceps femoral tendon; *SM* = soleus muscle; *GM* = gastrocnemius muscle (lateral head); *F* = fibula; *T* = tibia; *lat* = lateral aspect

KNEE POSTERIOR
Axial view
Popliteal fossa (Doppler)

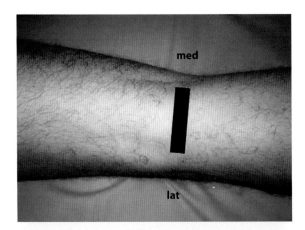

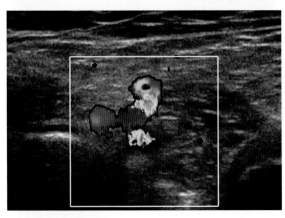
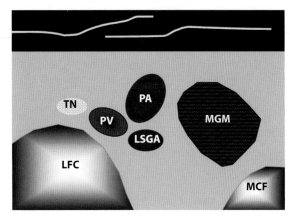

Fig. 2.65

Axial view of the popliteal fossa (color Doppler). *PA* = popliteal artery; *PV* = popliteal vein; *TN* = tibial nerve; *LSGA* = lateral superior geniculate artery; *LFC* = lateral femoral condyle; *MCF* = medial femoral condyle

ANKLE

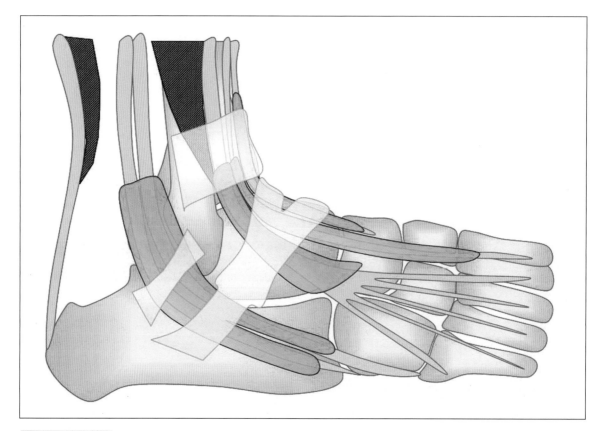

Fig. 2.66

Anatomical diagram of the ankle

ANKLE ANTERIOR
Longitudinal view
Anterior tibio-talar recess

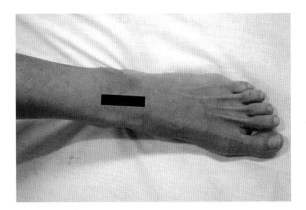

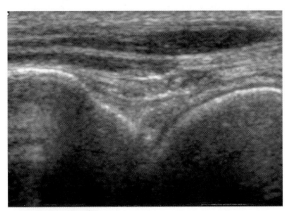 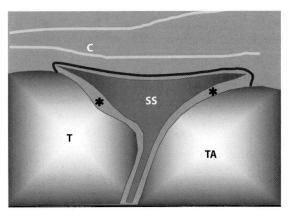

Fig. 2.67

Longitudinal scan of the anterior tibio-talar recess. *T* = tibia; *TA* = talus; *SS* = synovial space; *C* = capsule; * = articular cartilage

ANKLE ANTERIOR
Long axis view
Tibialis anterior tendon

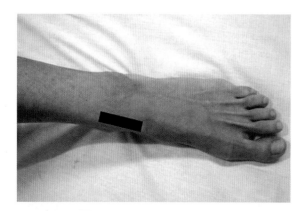

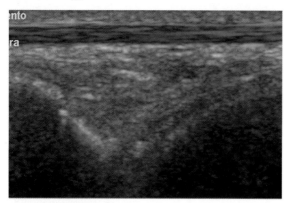
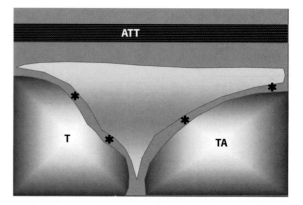

Fig. 2.68

Long axis view of the tibialis anterior tendon. *ATT* = tibialis anterior tendon; *T* = tibia; *TA* = talus; * = articular cartilage

ANKLE ANTERIOR
Axial view
Extensor tendons

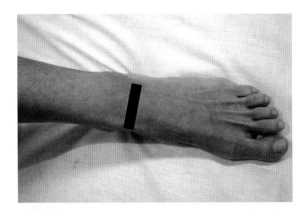

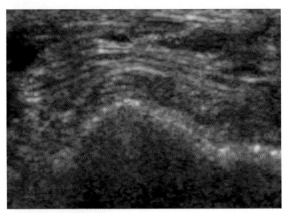
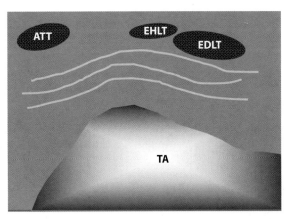

Fig. 2.69

Axial view of the anterior aspect of the ankle. *ATT* = anterior tibial tendon; *EHLT* = extensor hallucis longus tendon; *EDLT* = extensor digitorum longus tendon; *TA* = talus

ANKLE LATERAL
Long axis view
Anterior talo-fibular ligament

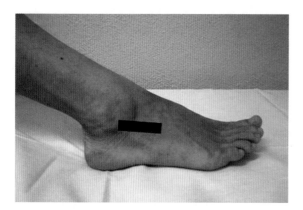

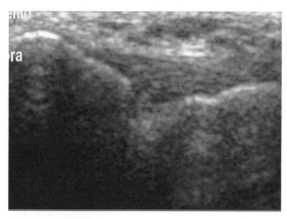

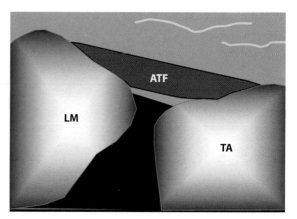

Fig. 2.70

Longitudinal view of anterior talo-fibular ligament. *ATF* = anterior talo-fibular ligament; *LM* = lateral malleolus; *TA* = talus

ANKLE LATERAL
Long axis view
Calcaneo-fibular ligament

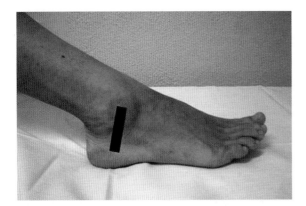

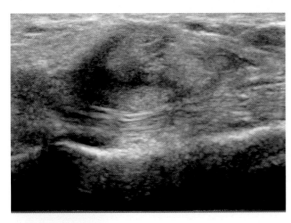

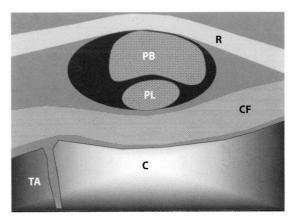

Fig. 2.71

Longitudinal view of the calcaneo-fibular ligament. *PB* = peroneus brevis; *PL* = peroneus longus; *CF* = calcaneo-fibular ligament; *C* = calcaneus; *TA* = talus; *R* = retinaculum

ANKLE LATERAL
Short axis view
Peroneal tendons

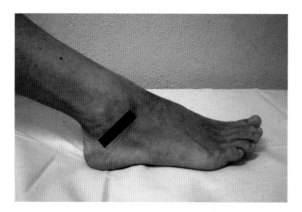

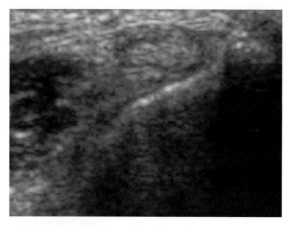
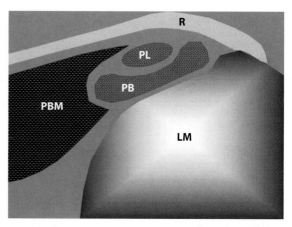

Fig. 2.72

Short axis view of the peroneal tendons. *PBM* = peroneus brevis muscle; *PB* = peroneus brevis; *PL* = peroneus longus; *R* = retinaculum; *LM* = lateral malleulus

ANKLE MEDIAL
Axial view
Tarsal tunnel

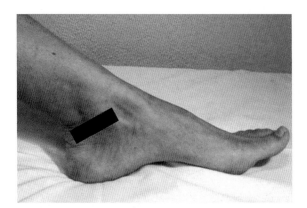

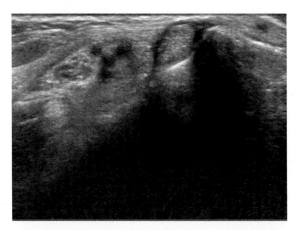
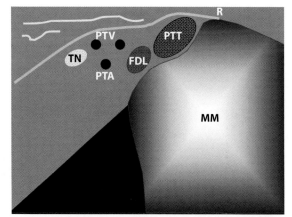

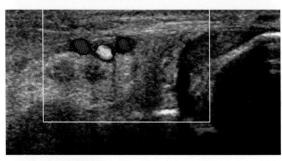
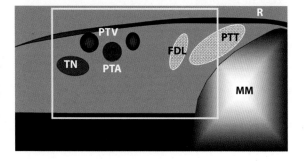

Fig. 2.73

Axial view of the medial aspect of the ankle. *TN* = posterior tibial nerve; *PTV* = posterior tibial veins; *PTA* = posterior tibial artery; *R* = retinaculum; *MM* = medial malleolus; *PTT* = posterior tibial tendon; *FDL* = flexor digitorum longus tendon

ANKLE MEDIAL
Long axis view
Deltoid ligament

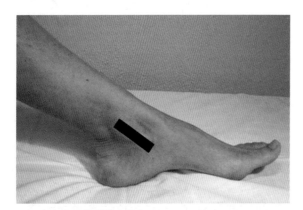

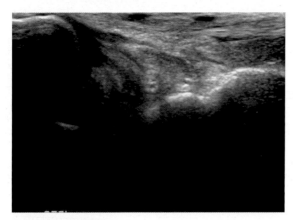

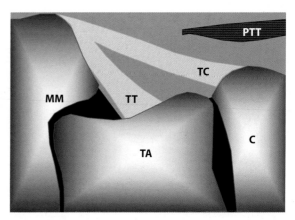

Fig. 2.74

Longitudinal view of deltoid ligament. *PTT* = posterior tibial tendon; *TC* = tibio-calcanear ligament; *TT* = tibio-talar ligament; *TA* = talus; *C* = calcaneus; *MM* = medial malleolus

ANKLE POSTERIOR
Long axis view
Achilles tendon

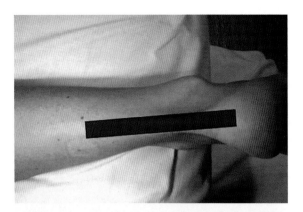

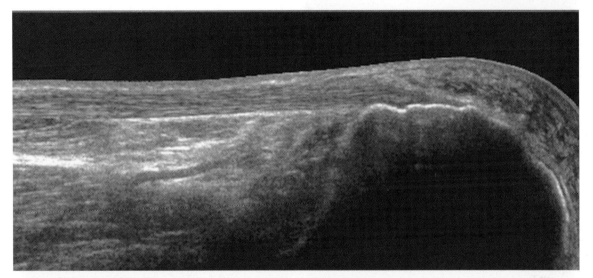

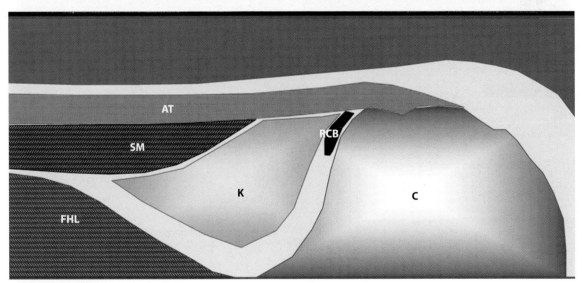

Fig. 2.75

Long axis view of the Achilles tendon. *AT* = Achilles tendon; *C* = calcaneus; *RCB* = retrocalcaneal bursa; *SM* = soleus muscle; *FHL* = flexor hallucis longus muscle; *K* = Kager soft pad

ANKLE POSTERIOR
Short axis view
Achilles tendon

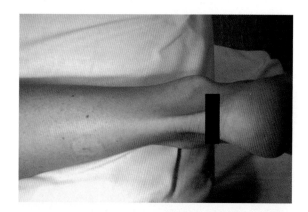

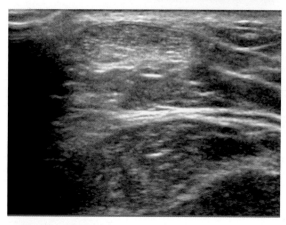

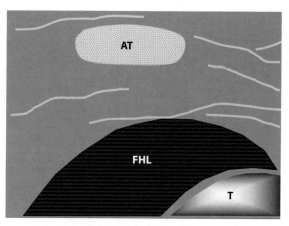

Fig. 2.76

Short axis view of the Achilles tendon. *AT* = Achilles tendon; *FHL* = flexor hallucis longus muscle; *T* = tibia

FOOT PLANTAR
Longitudinal view
Plantar fascia

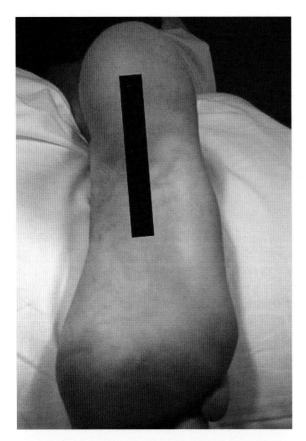

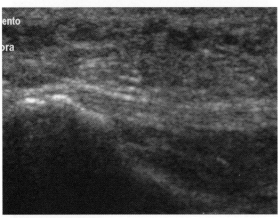

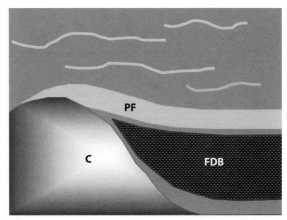

Fig. 2.77

Longitudinal view of the plantar fascia. *PF* = plantar fascia; *C* = calcaneus; *FDB* = flexor digitorum brevis muscle

FOOT PLANTAR
Longitudinal view
Metatarso-phalangeal joint

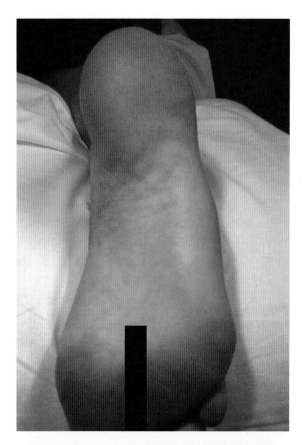

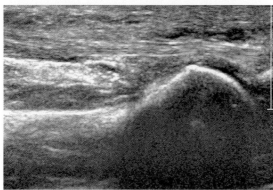

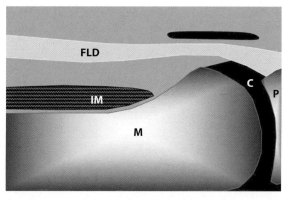

Fig. 2.78

Longitudinal view of the foot (metatarso-phalangeal joint). *FLD* = flexor longus digitorum tendon; *C* = capsule and synovial recess; *M* = metatarsal bone; *P* = phalanx; *IM* = interosseus muscle

FOOT PLANTAR
Axial view
Inter-metatarsal space

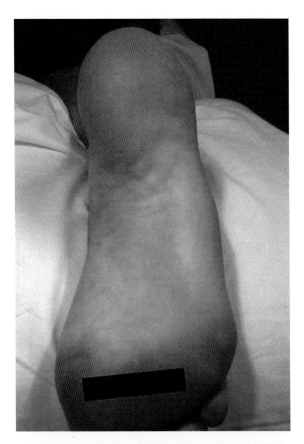

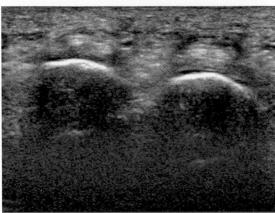

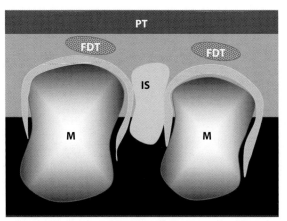

Fig. 2.79

Axial view of the foot. *M* = metatarsal bone; *FDT* = flexor digitorum tendon; *IS* = inter-metatarsal space; *PT* = plantar soft tissue

Sonographic and power Doppler normal anatomy

3.1 Cartilage

Cartilage is a greatly specialized type of connective tissue, mainly composed of water (70-80% by wet weight). It is avascular and aneural. The solid component of cartilage is formed of cells (chondrocytes) that are scattered in a firm gel-like substance (extracellular matrix) consisting of collagen and proteoglycans. Collagen forms a network of fibrils, which resists the swelling pressure generated by the proteoglycans. In the musculoskeletal system there are two types of cartilage: hyaline and fibrocartilage. Compared to hyaline, fibrocartilage contains more collagen and is more resistant at tensile strength. Fibrocartilage is found in intervertebral disks, symphyses, glenoid labra, menisci, the round ligament of the femur, and at sites connecting tendons or ligaments to bones. Hyaline cartilage is the most common variety of cartilage. It is found in costal cartilage, epiphyseal plates and covering bones in joints (articular cartilage). The free surfaces of most hyaline cartilage (but not articular cartilage) are covered by a layer of fibrous connective tissue (perichondrium). Hyaline cartilage structure is not uniform (Fig. 3.1). Instead, it is stratified and divided into four zones: superficial, middle, deep, and calcified. The superficial zone, also called **tangential zone**, is considered the articular surface and is characterized by flattened chondrocytes, relatively low quantities of proteoglycan, and numerous thicker fibrils arranged parallel to the articular surface in order to resist tension. In articular cartilage this layer acts as a barrier because there is no perichondrium. The middle zone, or **transitional zone**, in contrast, has round chondrocytes, the highest level of proteoglycan among the four zones, and a random arrangement of collagen. The deep (**radiate zone**) is the thickest zone, characterized by collagen fibrils that are perpendicular to the underlying bone, acting as an anchor to prohibit separation of zones and in order to resist at torsional and compressive mechanical strength. Columns of chondrocytes are arrayed along the axis of fibril orientation. The **zone of calcified cartilage** is partly mineralized, and acts as the transition between cartilage and the underlying subchondral bone. A boundary point (**tidemark**) represents a change in cartilage stiffness from radiate to calcified. The orientation of collagen fibers varies through the four zones of articular cartilage in order to give better tensile strength. The fibrillar framework seems to have an arcade-like arrangement, as hypothesized by Benninghoff. Nevertheless, the arcade model of Benninghoff has not been confirmed at electron microscopy evaluation.

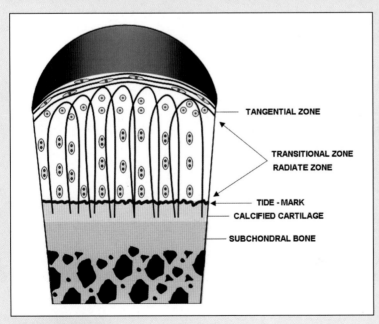

TANGENTIAL ZONE

TRANSITIONAL ZONE
RADIATE ZONE

TIDE - MARK
CALCIFIED CARTILAGE

SUBCHONDRAL BONE

Fig. 3.1

Anatomical diagram of hyaline cartilage structure

Hyaline cartilage is easily detectable by ultrasonography as a homogeneously hypo-anechoic layer delimited by thin, sharp and hyperechoic margins.

Normal articular cartilage appears as a well-defined layer with the following distinguishing features [1-3]:

1. high degree of homogeneous transparency due to its high water content;
2. sharp and continuous synovial space-cartilage interface (superficial margin);
3. sharp hyperechoic profile of the bone-cartilage interface (deep margin).

The synovial space-cartilage interface is slightly thinner than the bone-cartilage interface. Both margins are best visualized when the direction of the ultrasound (US) beam is perpendicular to the cartilage surface.

The pronounced difference in chemical structure between articular cartilage and subchondral bone allows easy detection of the deep margin, whilst the superficial margin requires careful examination techniques for clear identification.

Optimization of the visualization of the cartilage margins is essential for measuring the cartilage thickness [4].

Cartilage thickness ranges from 0.1 mm on the articular surface of the head of the proximal phalanx to 2.6 mm on the lateral femoral condyle of the knee joint [5]. Measurement of cartilage thickness is rapid (several seconds), painless, non-invasive and reproducible (inter-observer reproducibility of measurements of cartilage thickness seems to be relatively good) [6-8].

Sharp margins and homogeneity of the echotexture are hallmarks of normal cartilage (Figs. 3.2, 3.3).

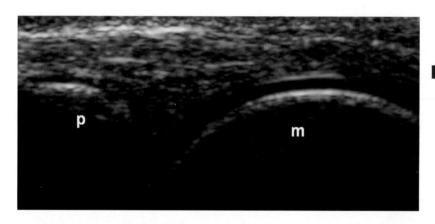

Fig. 3.2

Healthy subject. Longitudinal dorsal US scan of the second metacarpo-phalangeal joint obtained with a 5-13 MHz broadband linear transducer. The articular cartilage of the metacarpal head appears as a homogeneous anechoic layer with clearly defined hyperechoic contours. m = metacarpal head; p = proximal phalanx

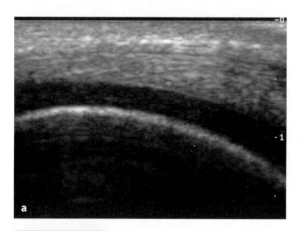

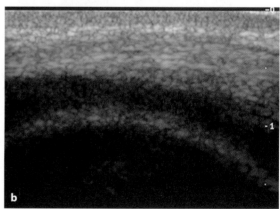

Fig. 3.3 a, b

Healthy subject. Knee. Suprapatellar longitudinal scan of the articular cartilage of the lateral femoral condyle obtained with a 5-10 MHz broadband linear transducer. **a** Normal features of the articular cartilage obtained with the ultrasound beam directly perpendicular to the cartilage surface. **b** Apparent loss of sharpness of the cartilage margins due to imperfect insonation angle

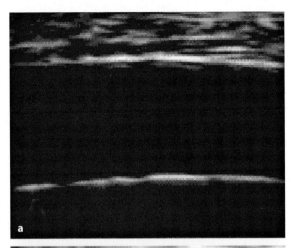

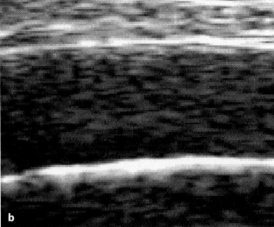

Fig. 3.4 a, b

Healthy subject. Knee. Suprapatellar longitudinal scan of the articular cartilage of the lateral femoral condyle obtained with an 8-16 MHz broadband linear transducer. Both images show the characteristic homogeneous echotexture of the cartilage layer. **a** Anechoic, obtained with low levels of gain. **b** Hypoechoic, obtained with relatively higher levels of gain

These sonographic features are remarkably similar at different anatomic sites and largely dependent upon the equipment settings.

The typical anechoic pattern is obtained at lower levels of gain (Fig. 3.4 a, b).

Many different factors contribute to the final sonographic visualization of the hyaline cartilage, including size of the acoustic window, operator experience, transducer frequency and patient position. In order to reduce misinterpretation, multiplanar examination and comparison with the contra-lateral side must be carried out [2, 9].

The complex anatomical structure of the knee joint poses particular acoustic barriers to accurate evaluation of the cartilage, meaning that only femoral condylar cartilage can be assessed.

The weight-bearing surfaces of the femoral condyles can be assessed by transverse suprapatellar scanning with the knee in maximal flexion or with an infrapatellar transverse scan with the leg fully extended.

Suprapatellar scanning of weight-bearing areas can be difficult in patients with limited degrees of flexion due to pain.

Further assessment of the weight-bearing cartilage of the medial femoral condyle can also be obtained by the medial parapatellar view with the knee in maximal flexion.

The transverse suprapatellar scan of the knee demonstrates that, in healthy subjects, the femoral cartilage typically appears as a clear-cut, wavy hypoanechoic layer, with upper concavity, which is thicker at the level of the intercondyloid fossa (Fig. 3.5).

This particular scan should be carried out with the knee flexed to an angle of at least 90°. A panoramic view of the entire cartilaginous profile can best

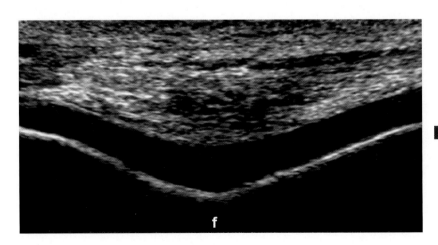

Fig. 3.5

Healthy subject. Suprapatellar transverse view of the knee. Articular cartilage appears as a curved anechoic band. The image was obtained with an Aplio, Toshiba, equipped with a 7-14 MHz broadband linear transducer. f = femur

be obtained with wide footprint and medium frequency probes (not higher than 10 MHz). Linear probes do not allow the ultrasound beam to reach the cartilaginous layer with the same angle of incidence, leading to apparent inhomogeneity in the cartilaginous echotexture and profile of the margins.

In addition, the transverse scan demonstrates the femoral cartilage most clearly at the level of the peripheral portions of the femoral condyles.

Conversely, longitudinal scans carried out on contiguous planes allow for accurate evaluation of the profile of the condylar cartilage, from its most proximal portions that articulate with the patella, to the more distal portions that relate to the tibial plateau (Fig. 3.3).

Articular cartilage of the metacarpal head can be evaluated by longitudinal and transverse dorsal scans with the metacarpophalangeal joint held in maximal flexion. Standard longitudinal dorsal and volar scans also may be useful.

Higher frequency probes (> 10 MHz), must be used in order to study the articular cartilage of the metacarpal head. Particular attention must be paid to the identification of the superficial margin that, in healthy subjects, appears as a thin hyperechoic line (of about a tenth of a millimeter thick), visible in tracts perpendicular to the direction of the ultrasound beam. This must be identified in order to obtain a correct measurement of the cartilaginous thickness. In a healthy subject, the thickness of the cartilage of the metacarpal head can vary between 0.2 and 0.5 mm [10].

3.2 Synovial cavity and articular capsule

The synovial cavity (Fig. 3.6) is the space found between bone segments and articular capsule; it is delimited by a fibrous wrap internally covered by a synovial membrane and contains a slight film of synovial fluid. The synovial cavity consists, depending on where it is found, of the joint cavity, the bursae and the tendon sheaths [11].

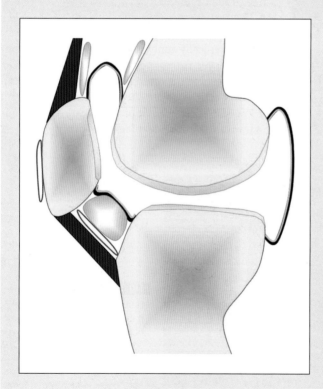

Fig. 3.6

Anatomical diagram of a synovial joint. Insertion and development of the articular capsule with the synovial membrane, articular cartilage and cavity, fat pads and bursae clearly shown

The **synovial fluid** has a variable volume according to the dimension of the articular cavity and it represents, physiologically, a thin veil to protect the cartilage surface; it acts as a lubricant and it has nourishing functions for the cartilage itself. The synovial fluid is filtered from the blood plasma and it contains a maximum of 200 cell/cc. It also contains electrolytes, glucose, enzymes, immunoglobulins and proteins mainly originating from blood, with the addition of *mucin* - mostly *hyaluronic acid* - which is well-represented. The mucin makes the synovial fluid viscous, elastic and plastic [12, 13].

The **articular capsule** consists of intertwisted bundles of connective fibrous tissue, whose insertion onto bone occurs as a continuous line. At some points the capsule is strengthened by the intrinsic capsular ligaments, represented by local thickenings (made of fibrous or fibro-elastic tissue) of the capsule itself, where the fiber bundles become parallel. The articular capsule is internally covered by the **synovial membrane**. The synovial membrane is a connective tissue of mesenchymal origin, covering any exposed osseous surface, the synovial bursae in communication with the joint cavity and the intracapsular ligament and tendons; it is not present on meniscal and discal surfaces and it stops right before the edge of joint cartilage, the peripheral area of which, only a few millimeters thick, constitutes a zone of transition from synovial membrane to cartilage [14].

In the synovial cavities of some joints, adipose tissue is stored in specific regions, forming mobile and elastic pads that fill in the spaces of the articular cavity. Such adipose stores, when the joint moves, adapt to the changes of shape and volume of the synovial cavity, supporting the lubrication of the joint surfaces.

The synovial membrane is made of a cellular intima lying on a fibrovascular subintimal lamina consisting of abundant loose areolar tissue, collagen and elastic fibers. When the synovial membrane covers the intracapsular tendons or ligaments, the subintima is hardly identifiable as a separate layer, being fused together with the capsule, the ligament or the adjacent tendon [12, 14].

The synovial intima is made of cells, called synoviocytes A and B, whose function is to remove the debris found in the joint cavity and to synthesize some molecules for the synovial fluid. The synoviocytes do not actively proliferate under basal conditions, while the speed of cellular division is considerably increased after trauma and acute hemarthrosis [13].

The **bursae** are virtual spaces localized in specific regions of the joint where high friction between closely opposing structures occurs. The bursae can be visualized almost solely in pathologic conditions, because they physiologically contain a slight film of synovial fluid. As above, the bursae are covered by the synovial membrane that continues from the synovial membrane of the articular cavity, so that it constitutes communicating bursae where the synovial fluid is freely circulating. The communicating bursae have a further biomechanical function: they decrease the endoarticular pressure when there is a fluid collection in the joint cavity.

Normally, the synovial cavities are barely or invisible with US, whereas they can be easily evaluated when a thickening of the synovial membrane or a joint fluid collection occurs. The size of the synovial cavity of the **hip** can be depicted and measured by US using a sagittal view passing through the femoral head – the lower limb externally rotated 10-15°; in healthy subjects the interposed distance between the femoral neck outline and the articular capsule has a mean value of 5.1 mm (range 3-7 mm). There is no evident relationship between the sono-graphic size of the synovial cavity and age, gender, height or body weight; the maximum difference between one side and the contralateral side is about 1 mm.

In the **knee**, the only synovial cavity accessible to US is the suprapatellar recess. The examination can be performed through supra-patellar longitudinal and axial views, with the patient lying supine with the knee in the extended position. The suprapatellar recess appears as a hypoechoic flat structure, with a regular and clear contour, whose antero-posterior diameter does not measure more than 3-4 millimeters.

Dynamic assessment, performed during contraction of the quadriceps femoris muscle, shows a slight increase both in the antero-posterior diameter and in the recess length.

The increase in fluid collection during this phase, related to the mean sagittal diameter increase of the bursa (1 mm), can be related to the simultaneous contraction of the suprapatellar recess tensor muscle. This small muscle drags the bursa, causing a vacuum effect that causes the bursa to fill with fluid coming from the joint cavity [4]. In people who are fit, compared to those who lead a sedentary life, the suprapatellar recess diameter does not change, but it is well-visualized in 25% and in 66% of patients, respectively, according to the relaxation and the contraction of the quadriceps femoris [15].

The synovial membrane contour can be indirectly assessed when the suprapatellar recess is distended by synovial fluid. It appears as a thin echoic band of 1.7 mm (mean value) [4]. The anterior synovial layer of the suprapatellar recess is usually more easily identified than the deep layer. The first can be easily assessed thanks to the different echogenicity of the overlying quadriceps tendon, which appears moderately echoic, while the latter is strictly contiguous with the pre-femoral fat pad, which is echoic and has a maximum thickness of about 1 cm. Normally the synovial fluid in the subquadricipital recess is homogeneously hypoanechoic and any change is related to pathology (Fig. 3.7).

The **articular capsule**, is extremely thin and can be barely identified by ultrasound in physiological situations, whereas acute, inflammatory, or post-traumatic pathology makes it easily visible because of the natural acoustic window provided by the joint fluid collection.

In order to identify the capsule, it is necessary to have precise anatomical reference points, joint by joint.

The articular capsule appears as a thin hyperechoic layer, hard to differentiate from the adjacent tendons and ligaments that have very similar echogenicity [16].

In the shoulder, the superior edge of the capsule corresponds to the inferior echoic edge of the tendons of the rotator cuff muscles (supraspinatus, infraspinatus and teres minor); it is only when pathology occurs, such as an adhesive capsulitis – causing thickening and retraction – that the capsule can be identified as a marked irregularity of the inferior profile of the rotator cuff tendons. The axillary recess of the inferior edge of the capsule is more easily explored.

The articular capsule of the knee can be easily assessed in the internal and external compartments, where the collateral ligaments delineate the capsule borders. The same procedure can be applied to assess any other joint of the hand and foot [16, 17].

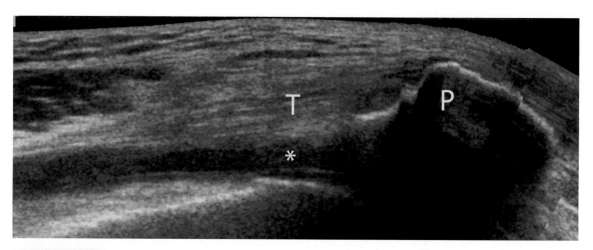

Fig. 3.7

Longitudinal extended field of view (EFV) US scan of anterior compartment of the knee. Small amount of fluid in the joint (*) and distension of suprapatellar capsular recess. T = quadriceps tendon; P = patella

3.3 Tendons, adnexa, and ligaments

Tendons are critical biomechanical units in the musculoskeletal system, the function of which is to transmit the muscular tension to mobile skeletal segments. They are extremely resistant to traction, almost like bone. A tendon with a 10 mm² transverse section can bear a maximum of 600-1000 kg. On the other hand, tendons are not very elastic, and can only tolerate a maximum elongation of 6% before being damaged.

Tendons have very slow metabolism, even during action. This can be significantly increased only by inflammatory conditions and traumas. When a reparative process occurs, a proliferation of fibrocytes is observed with deposition of collagen cells [18, 19].

Tendons macroscopically appear as ribbon-like structures, with extremely variable shape and dimensions, characterized by the presence of dense fibrous tissue arranged in parallel bundles. More specifically, they consist of about 70% of type I collagen fibers that form primary bundles. Among the primary bundles are fibrocytes endowed with large laminar protrusions, named tenocytes or alar cells. Among the collagen fibers of tendons, elastic fibers (about 4%) can also be found; their role is not different from that of a "shock absorber" when muscular contraction begins. The collagen and elastic fibers both have the same direction as the main lines of force and are lying in a gel consisting of proteoglycans and water. The **primary bundles** are assembled to form **secondary bundles** (representing the tendon's functional unit), which are clustered in **tertiary bundles**.

The **endotenon** is a thin connective strip surrounding the primary, secondary and tertiary bundles, and separating them. Vessels and nerves run within the endotenon thickness. The **epitenon** is a stronger connective covering, surrounding the whole tendon (Fig. 3.8) [14, 20].

From a functional and anatomical point of view, tendons can be divided into two types: *supporting tendons* (or anchor tendons) and *sliding tendons*.

Anchor tendons (such as the Achilles and the patellar tendon) are typically bigger and stronger than sliding tendons, they are not provided with a synovial sheath, but they are surrounded by a connective lamina external to the epitenon, called **peritenon**; the two connective sheaths (epitenon and peritenon) form the **paratenon** together with highly vascularized adipose and areolar tissue [20].

Sliding tendons are wrapped in a covering sheath (**tenosynovial sheath**) whose function is to guarantee better sliding and protection to the tendons when they run adjacent to irregular osseous surfaces, sites of potential friction. The tenosynovial sheath consists of two layers: a visceral layer, strictly con-

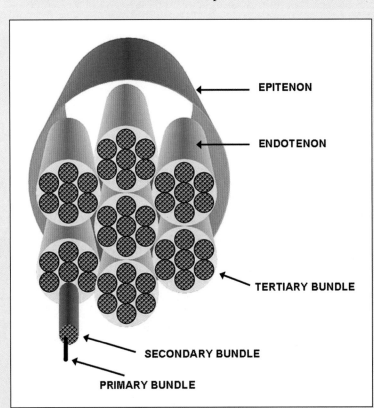

EPITENON

ENDOTENON

TERTIARY BUNDLE

SECONDARY BUNDLE

PRIMARY BUNDLE

Fig. 3.8

Anatomical drawing of a tendon

tiguous to the epitenon, and a parietal, more external, layer; the two layers come together to form a synovial "fold" named **mesotenon**. A closed cavity, nearly virtual, containing a very small amount of synovial fluid, is found between the two layers (Fig. 3.9) [14, 19, 20].

The tenosynovial sheath of sliding tendons corresponds anatomically and functionally to the peritenon of anchor tendons and, similarly, the tenosynovial sheath and the epitenon together constitute the paratenon of the sliding tendon [14].

The *vascularization* varies according to the type of tendon. In sliding tendons, the vessels run within the mesotenon, the mentioned synovial "fold" which connects the parietal and visceral layers. The vessels pass therefore along the tendon's surface, where some arterioles arising from the vessels penetrate into the tendon following the course of connective laminae (Fig. 3.10).

On the other hand, the vessels of the anchor tendons constitute a thick and irregular anastomotic net within the paratenon. Arteriolar vessels arise from this net and penetrate inside the tendon to different levels, following the course of the connective laminae. The arterioles, within these connective structures, form vascular arcades with the nearby arterioles [21].

Tendons may present with less vascularized zones, named **critical areas**, which are extremely important in the pathogenesis of several tendon diseases. Examples include the pre-insertional area of the supraspinatus tendon of the shoulder, or the central part of the Achilles tendon, which typically constitute highly susceptible sites of degenerative disease and tendon rupture.

The points of union between the tendons and the muscle or the bone are named myotendinous junction and osteotendinous junction (enthesis), respectively. The **myotendinous junction** is usually well-defined: at this level the tendon fibers are intertwined with the endomysium fibers. The **osteotendinous junction** has a more complicated structure: its nature may be either fibrous or fibrocartilaginous according to the tendon mobility, the angle formed between the tendon fibers and the bone, and the presence of an underlying retinaculum. The tendons moving in a single spatial plan and whose insertion on the bone occurs with an acute angle (for example, the flexor tendons of the toes), have a fibrous enthesis. The same situation occurs for tendons whose course is modified and kept in position by a retinaculum – for example the peroneal tendons – and whose insertion on the bone once again forms an acute angle.

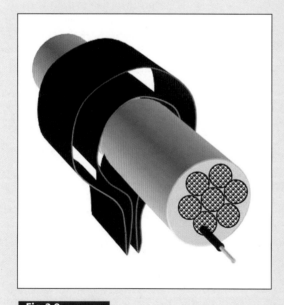

Fig. 3.9

Anatomical pattern of a tendon sheath

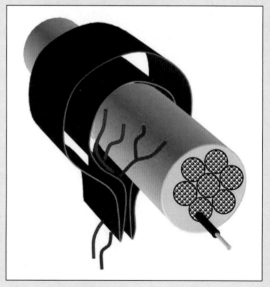

Fig. 3.10

Vascularization of a sliding tendon. Vessels arise from mesotenon

The tendons controlling multiplanar movement (for example the Achilles tendon) and whose insertion on the bone surface is orthogonal, have a thick fibro-cartilaginous enthesis that minimizes the risk of tendon tear. This more complicated type of osteotendinous junction consists of four layers in quick succession, represented - from the most superficial to the deepest one - by tendinous tissue, fibrocartilage, calcified fibrocartilage and bone. The osteotendinous junction is well-vascularized and the paratenon vascular net is anastomosed with that of the periostium [14, 20, 21].

A retinaculum is a transversal thickening of the deep fascia attached to a bone's eminence.

The biomechanical function of a retinaculum is to keep the tendons in position as they pass underneath it, in order to avoid their dislocation during muscular action. Retinacula therefore guarantee that tendons are correctly deviated and kept in position in their respective osteofibrous canals, allowing their efficient action; the synovial sheath, which always covers these types of tendons, makes the sliding of a tendon easy, and reduces friction. Retinacula are typically found in the wrist and ankle.

Some examples are the transverse carpal ligament, which defines the superior aspect of the carpal tunnel, where the flexor digitorum tendons and the median nerve run, and the ankle retinacula, which stabilize the flexor and extensor tendons in their deflexion points [22].

Some specific types of retinacula are found in the fingers, where the flexor digitorum tendons, wrapped in the synovial sheath, run along osteofibrous canals extending from the palm of the hand to the distal phalanx. The superior aspect of these osteofibrous canals (the "vault") consists of arch-like fibers running over the tendons, in points where more stabilization is needed.

For their peculiar biomechanical function, these structures are named **flexor annular pulleys**.

On the contrary, in regions where the canal needs to be more flexible, in order to allow the flexion of joints, a device consisting of loose plaited fibers is present, providing support to the tendon sheath without fixing it [23].

Ligaments have an analogous structure to that of tendons; however, they are thinner and they contain a higher amount of elastin, which is a necessary element to supply these structures with some degree of elasticity for their very important biomechanical role in the stabilization of joints. There are two types of ligaments: the intrinsic capsular ligaments, which appear as localized thickenings within the capsule with a strengthening function, and the extrinsic ligaments, which are independent from the fibrous capsule and can be further classified as extracapsular and intracapsular ligaments [14, 23].

Nowadays US represents the gold standard technique for the assessment of tendons [24, 25]. With the advent, for clinical purposes, of high resolution transducers and specific image processing software, it became possible to make detailed analysis of the shape and structure of tendons. In addition, US is the only technique that allows the radiologist to perform a dynamic study of tendons, which is extremely important for the diagnosis of tendon pathology. In longitudinal ultrasound views (long axis), the tendons appear as echoic ribbon-like bands, defined by a marginal hyperechoic line corresponding to the paratenon and characterized by a fibrillar internal structure. The fibrillar echotexture is represented by a succession of thin hyperechoic parallel bands, slightly wavy, which tend to grow apart from one another when the tendon is released and to move closer when the tendon is tense. This fibrillar echostructure is caused by the specular reflections within the tendon determined by the existing acoustic interface between the endotenon septa

(Fig. 3.11). The number and thickness of such structures change depending on the frequency of the transducer [26]. In transversal views (short axis), tendons appear as round or oval-shaped structures, characterized by several homogeneously scattered spotty echoes (Fig. 3.12).

In transverse views the Achilles tendon thickness (antero-posterior diameter) can be best assessed. In transverse section the Achilles tendon is elliptical, with its major axis following an oblique antero-medial direction. The sonographer must be aware of the risk of overestimating tendon thickness when assessed on longitudinal scans [24, 26].

When evaluating a tendon by US, it is extremely important to apply a correct orthogonal direction to the US beam, both for longitudinal and axial

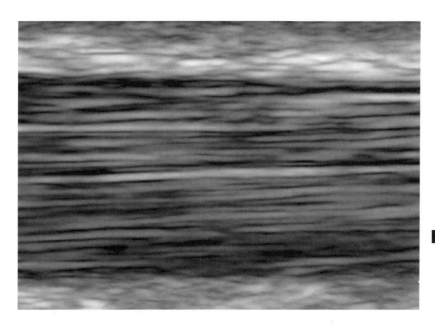

Fig. 3.11

The fibrillar echotexture of a normal tendon is created by the interfaces between collagen fibers and endotenon septa (long axis scan)

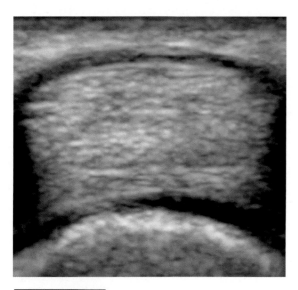

Fig. 3.12

Short axis sonogram showing the characteristic hyperechoic pattern, with scattered spotty echoes

views. When the US beam is not orthogonal to the tendon course, both a decrease of the reflected echoes and an increase of the diffracted ones occur, resulting in a significant or partial reduction of the tendon echotexture (tendon anisotropy) [26]. This artifact is more frequently found when assessing the rotator cuff tendons of the shoulder, the quadriceps femoris, the patellar and Achilles tendons, the osteotendinous junctions, the flexor and extensor tendons of the ankle, hand and wrist. In these regions a less experienced sonographer can risk making an incorrect diagnosis (Fig. 3.13) [26].

The sliding and anchor tendons present some differences regarding their US appearance. Sliding tendons, as already described, are wrapped in a synovial sheath which contains, even in physiological situations, a minimum amount of synovial fluid acting as a lubricant. This slight film of fluid can be easily recognized, both in axial views and in longitudinal views, as a thin anechoic halo sur-

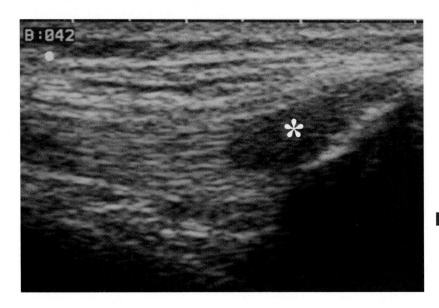

Fig. 3.13

Longitudinal US scan of relaxed quadriceps tendon in a healthy man. The hypoechoic spot (*) (tendon anisotropy) corresponds to the pre-insertional area

rounding the tendon. The pathological increase in synovial fluid inside the tendon sheath often allows the mesotenon to be identified.

On the other hand, anchor tendons are surrounded by the peritenon, a layer of dense connective tissue leaning on the epitenon, which contributes to constitute the paratenon. The paratenon appears as an echoic line surrounding the tendon, without the possibility of distinguishing, in normal conditions, between peritenon and epitenon [26, 28].

High resolution ultrasound is performed to study the inflammatory pathology of tendons in order to depict the morphological and structural variety of tendons and the synovial sheath expansion. The gray-scale ultrasound technique is still not able to recognize indirect signs of inflammation.

By implementing the information obtained from a gray-scale ultrasound examination with that obtained from a power Doppler study, the sonographer is able to identify functional parameters regarding the vascularization of the tendons for a better clinical evaluation.

In standard conditions, tendons have low metabolic activity and the blood supply is given by high resistance arteries and small veins, too thin to be studied with the Doppler technique.

In such cases, weak flow signals can be observed near small arterial structures afferent to the cortical bone. These vascular structures are usually arteries with a high resistance index, corresponding to the periosteal vessels [29].

Several conditions such as inflammatory, post-traumatic and infectious, are responsible for the activation of vascular hyperemia with an increase in blood flow and a drop in vascular resistance.

In this way the tendon vessels become easy to assess with color or power Doppler technique and it is also possible to perform a semiquantitative flow analysis of pulsed wave Doppler ultrasound spectrum (Fig. 3.14) [29].

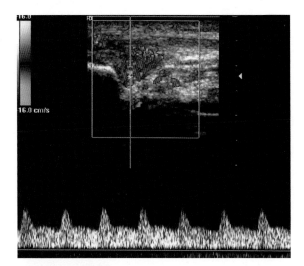

Fig. 3.14

Color Doppler scan in jumper's knee. Peri- and intratendinous hypervascularization of the proximal third of the tendon is clearly shown. The spectral analysis shows arteries with low resistance and high diastolic flow

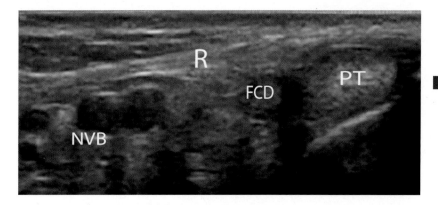

Fig. 3.15

Transverse US scan of the medial compartment of the ankle. The retinaculum (*R*) is the thin hyperechoic line that lies over the tendons. *PT* = posterior tibial; *CFD* = communis flexor digitorum, *NVB* = neurovascular bundle

Retinacula at ultrasound appear as thin hyperechoic structures located more superficially than the sliding tendons, in very critical areas from a biomechanical point of view (Fig 3.15). Annular *pulleys* are biomechanical devices made of fibrous connective tissue, which keep the flexor digitorum tendons in position during flexion-extension movements.

For this reason, the sonographic assessment of the pulleys has to be performed with a dynamic method; the US dynamic analysis should be obtained during flexion-extension movements of the fingers and, if a tendon tear is suspected, it should be supplemented with contrasted flexion. The transducer should always have a perpendicular and transverse position over the flexor tendons, with a high amount of gel used as a spacer in order to avoid any pressure on the tissue. In longitudinal views of flexor tendons, the pulley appears as a thin oval structure lying superficially compared with the tendon sheath (Fig. 3.16) [30, 31].

The structure of ***ligaments*** is very similar to that of tendons; the main differences are reduced thickness and a less regular arrangement of structural elements; for this reason, it is harder to study ligaments with US than tendons.

The US examination of ligaments, unlike tendons, is mainly performed using long axis views, the transducer being aligned on the ligament's major axis. Transverse views (short axis) have poor diagnostic value. With US, ligaments appear as homogeneous, hyperechoic bands, 2-3 mm thick, lying close to the bone (Fig 3.17) [32].

The easiest ligaments to assess with US are those of the medial and lateral compartments of the ankle (deltoid, anterior talofibular and fibulocalcaneal), the collateral ligaments of the knee, the collateral and annular ligaments of the elbow, the coraco-acromial and coraco-humeral ligaments of the shoulder and the ulnar collateral ligament of the thumb [30-32].

The medial collateral ligament of the knee (MCL) has a very complicated structure that deserves detailed description. The MCL is a flattened, large structure extending from the distal

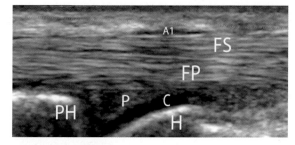

Fig. 3.16

Longitudinal US scan of flexor digitorum tendons at the metacarpophalangeal joint. The first (*A1*) out of five pulleys is clearly shown over the tendons. *FP* = flexor digitorum profundus; *FS* = flexor digitorum superficialis; *PH* = proximal phalanx; *H* = metacarpal head; *P* = palmar plate; *C* = cartilage

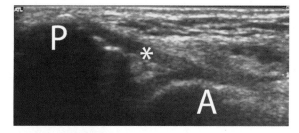

Fig. 3.17

Transverse US scan of the lateral compartment of the ankle. The anterior talo-fibular ligament (*) is tight between the anterior part of the lateral malleolus (*P*) and the talus (*A*)

extremity of the medial femoral condyle to the proximal tibial extremity; it is about 9 cm long and it is divided into two components, deep and superficial, which are separated by a thin layer of loose connective tissue. The deep component is then divided into two small ligaments that fix the medial meniscus respectively to the femur (meniscofemoral ligament) and to the tibia (menisco-tibial ligament). Sonographically the MCL appears as a trilaminar structure consisting of two hyperechoic layers, separated by a central interleaved hypoechoic area. The hyperechoic bands correspond to deep and superficial fiber bundles; whereas the loose areolar tissue constitutes the hypoechoic central area that divides the superficial component from the deep one (Fig. 3.18) [32].

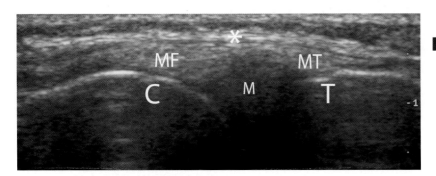

Fig. 3.18

Longitudinal US scan of the medial compartment of the knee. The complex structure of medial collateral ligament is shown. * = superficial portion, *MF* = meniscofemoral deep portion, *MT* = menisco-tibial deep portion; *C* = femoral condyle; *T* = tibial plateau; *M* = meniscus

3.4 Muscles

Muscle is made of bundles of contractile elementary units – **the striated muscle fibers** – with their major axis lying along the contraction direction. The muscular fibers are multinuclear cellular units derived, during embryonal development, from mesodermal cells of the primitive segments. The fibers have a cylindrical or polyhedral shape with smoothed angles; they have a considerable length, varying from a few millimeters to several centimeters, and a width between 10 and 100 mm. Considerable differences between different muscle fibers can be observed and, even within the same muscle, the fibers' diameter can vary according to work, nutritional conditions and other causes.

Muscular fibers are arranged parallel to one another and they are supported by a structure of connective tissue. Muscle is externally surrounded by a thick connective sheath called the **epimysium**; from the internal aspect of this sheath several septa depart to constitute the **perimysium**, which surrounds diverse bundles of muscular fibers, named **fascicles**. Blood vessels and nerves run within the perimysium, which also contains the neuromuscular spindles. Very light and thin septa arising from the perymysium spread into the fascicles to surround every single muscular fiber and thus form the **endomysium**. The endomysium, a network made of reticular fibers, blood capillaries, a few connective cells together with some small nervous bundles, constitutes the framework found right around the striated muscle fibers, and it represents the site of metabolic exchange between striated muscle fibers and blood (Fig. 3.19) [14, 23, 33].

The epimysial, perimysial and endomysial coverings come together where muscles connect to adjacent structures: the extremity of the muscle may continue as a tendon or insert onto the periosteum, aponeurosis or the dermis; this structure is extremely resistant, since the tensile forces turn into tangential forces that are more easily born. At a submicroscopic level, the muscular fibers end in a conical shape and adapt to the connective tissue just like fingers adapt to a glove; at the two endpoints of the muscular fiber, the myofibrils are attached to the sarcolemma. By means of these devices, the muscular fibers are strongly connected to the terminal insertion and the force developed by contraction does not lose any efficiency at the passage from muscle to tendon and

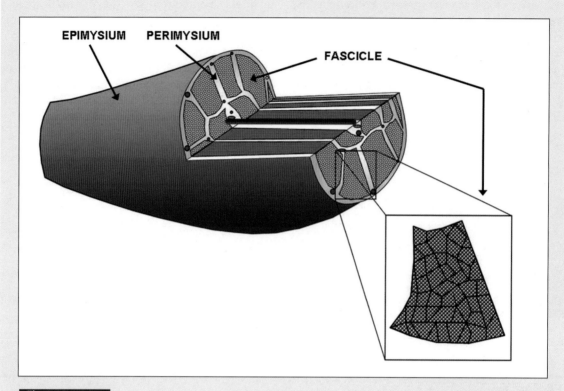

Fig. 3.19

Anatomical drawing of a muscle with magnification of a fascicle showing its endomysial framework

there is no risk of detachment. From a clinical point of view, such detachments occur only in rare situations, for it is much easier for a tendon to detach from a bone fragment at its insertion, in the case of an exceptionally strong contraction.

The macroscopic shape of muscles varies according to their function. Each muscle presents at least one muscular belly and two tendons, one at the origin and the other at the insertion. In some cases, like the rectus abdominis muscle, the muscle consists of different bellies united together with fibrous insertions. Another possible structure is observed for example in the biceps, triceps and quadriceps muscles, consisting of multiple origins and insertions on a single muscular belly.

The most frequent setting is the semipennate type for both extremities of the muscle. In this case, tendons are wide, flattened and oriented in the opposite direction, originating respectively from one side and the other of the muscle. The muscular bundles are directed from tendon to tendon and the shorter and more numerous they are, the wider the tendon insertion is. This setting influences the biomechanics, because the degree of muscular shortening depends on the fibers' length and the energy of contraction depends on the number of fibers constituting the muscle; two muscles with the same length, width and thickness, and therefore the same volume, but with different number and length of fibers, will also have different shortening capability and contraction energy. Therefore, when assessing the biomechanical characteristics of a muscle, not only the volume should be taken into account, but also the type of insertion, whose width influences the number and length of the fibers. The internal structure of skeletal muscle varies according to its specific function. Muscles with fibers parallel to the longitudinal axis (muscles of the abdomen, head and neck) are made for bearing reasonable weights for long distance activities. On the other hand, the uni-, bi- and circum-pennate settings (muscles of the limbs) can bear greater weights for a shorter period of time.

The internal structure of muscles can be easily assessed by ultrasound imaging. The external connective sheath of the muscle (epimysium) appears as a hyperechoic external band measuring a maximum of 2-3 mm of thickness and, on longitudinal US sections, continues without interruption along the corresponding tendon profile (Fig. 3.20).

The fibro-adipose septa (perimysium) are seen as hyperechoic lines separating the contiguous hypoechoic muscular bundles (fascicles) from one another (Fig. 3.21).

The typical pennate structure of muscles can be easily assessed in longitudinal axis views (Fig. 3.22 a), where the hyperechoic fibro-adipose septa converge, with a mainly parallel course, on a central aponeurosis, appearing as a thin, highly reflective band [32, 34].

Ultrasound evaluation of the direction of the muscle fibers represents an important parameter for the measurement of the pennation angle; this angle is measured between the muscular fibers' direction and the central aponeurosis axis (usually corresponding to the longitudinal muscular axis). The value of the angle varies depending on the function of the muscle and, within the same muscle, on the functional state (contraction/relaxation). In transverse views, the muscle is sectioned according to a plane that is orthogonal to the muscular longitudinal axis, with a typical US structure appearance; the 1st and 2nd order fascicles show an irregu-

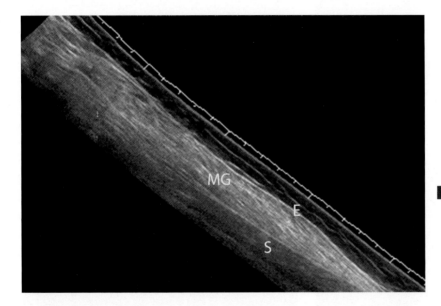

Fig. 3.20

EFV scan of the sural triceps. *MG* = medial gastrocnemius; *S* = soleus; *E* = epimysium. The hyperechoic appearance of the epimysium wrapping the muscle bellies and continuing to the aponeurosis is shown

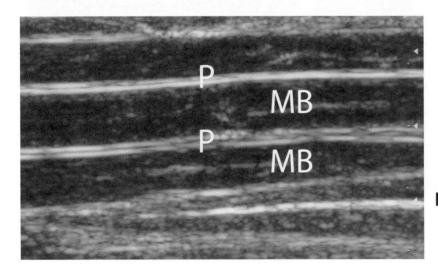

Fig. 3.21

'In vitro' scan of bovine muscle. The hyperechoic appearance of perimysial septa (*P*) wrapping the muscle bellies (*MB*) is shown

lar polygonal shape, defined by thin, elongated, hyperechoic septa corresponding to the perimysial fibro-adipose septa (Fig. 3.22 b) [32, 34, 35].

When studying both muscles and tendons, it is fundamental that the ultrasound beam is correctly tilted so that it is always perpendicular to the examined muscular plane, in order to avoid the appearance of hypoechoic artifactual zones

that can be misinterpreted by inexperienced operators [36, 37].

In some body regions the sonographer can observe accessory muscles, not to be misinterpreted as pathologic masses. The most common described "pseudomasses" are the palmaris longus muscle at the wrist [38], the accessory soleus and the peroneus quartus at the ankle.

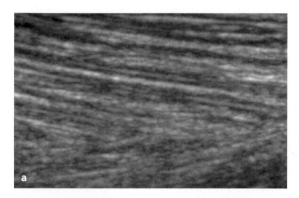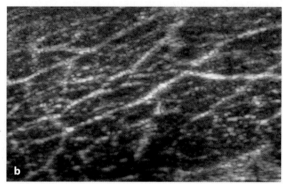

Fig. 3.22 a, b

a Longitudinal US scan of a pennate muscle. The characteristic pennate appearance is given by the convergence of perimysial septa.
b The transverse US scan shows the polygonal arrangement of the muscular fascicles and hyperechoic perimysial septa

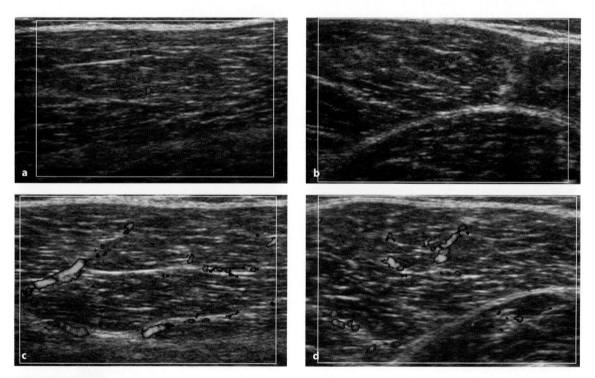

Fig. 3.23 a-d

Color Doppler longitudinal (**a**, **c**) and transverse (**b**, **d**) scans of the quadriceps (vastus lateralis) before (**a**, **b**) and after exercise (**c**, **d**). A diffuse intramuscular hypervascularization is shown after intense activity. This is related to the physiological hyperemia

US examination should always be performed as a comparative technique with the contralateral muscle and in an active and passive dynamic way, both during contraction and during relaxation. This allows a functional evaluation of the muscle.

The degree of muscular contraction affects the oblique direction of the echoic septal pattern; in particular a higher obliquity of the fibers is observed when the muscle is relaxed. The images obtained during an isometric contraction may show an apparent increase of the muscular mass and of the hypoechogenicity depending on the muscular bundles' thickening during contraction. Hypertrophy of the muscular bundles, typically observed in athletes, can be associated with increased muscular hypoechogenicity [39].

Finally, physical exercise is associated with an increase in muscular vascularization (blood flow is 20 times higher than in standard conditions) and a consequent increase in the muscular mass volume, up to 10-15%. The muscular volume gets back to standard conditions after about 10-15 minutes of rest [18].

Doppler techniques and, more specifically, power Doppler, can demonstrate the physiological muscular hyperemia after contraction (Fig. 3.23 a-d).

3.5 Nerves

From an anatomical point of view, nerves are characterized by a complex internal structure made of nervous fibers (containing axons, myelin sheaths and Schwann cells) grouped in fascicles, and loose connective tissue (containing elastic fibers and vessels) (Fig. 3.24 a). A closer look at nerve sheaths demonstrates an external sheath – the **outer epineurium** – which surrounds the **nerve fascicles**. Each fascicle is invested in turn with a proper connective sheath – the **perineurium** – which encloses a variable number of nerve fibers separated by the **endoneurium**. The connective tissue intervening between the outer nerve sheath and the fascicles is commonly referred to as the **interfascicular epineurium** and houses the nerve vasculature.

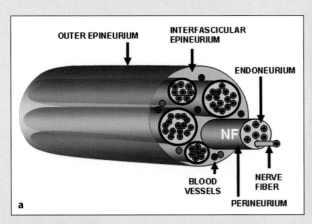
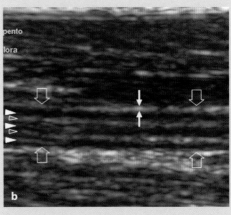

Fig. 3.24 a, b

Peripheral nerves. **a** Schematic drawing illustrating the inner structure of a peripheral nerve. *NF* = nerve fascicle. **b** Longitudinal 5-12 MHz US image obtained over the median nerve (*empty arrows*) at the middle third of the forearm. The nerve is composed of parallel linear hypoechoic areas (*white arrowheads*) - the fascicles - separated by hyperechoic bands (*empty arrowheads*) - the interfascicular epineurium. Note the outer epineurium (*white arrows*)

With the current generation of high-frequency "small parts" transducers and compound technology, US has become a well-accepted and widespread imaging modality for evaluation of peripheral nerves. The improved performance of these transducers has made it possible to recognize subtle anatomical details with US at least equal to or even smaller than those depicted with surface-coil magnetic resonance (MR) imaging and to depict a wide range of pathological conditions affecting nerves [40, 41]. Apart from the availability of high-end technology, nerve US requires indepth knowledge of anatomy and close correlation of imaging findings with the patient's clinical history and the results of electrophysiological studies. With these credentials, US provides low-cost and non-invasive imaging, speed of performance, and other important advantages over MR imaging, including a higher spatial resolution and the ability to explore long segments of nerve trunks in a single study and to examine nerves in both static and dynamic states with real time scanning.

On long axis planes, nerves typically assume an elongated appearance with multiple hypoechoic parallel linear areas, which correspond to the neuronal fascicles that run longitudinally within the nerve, separated by hyperechoic bands [42] (Fig. 3.24 b). On short axis planes, high-resolution US demonstrates nerves as honeycomb-like structures composed of hypoechoic rounded areas (the fascicles) embedded in a hyperechoic background (interfascicular epineurium) (Fig. 3.25 a, b) [42].

The number of fascicles in a nerve may vary depending on the occurrence of nerve branching. In nerve bifurcations, the nerve trunk divides into two or more secondary nerve bundles, whereas each fascicle enters only one of the divisional branches without splitting. The outer boundaries of nerves are usually undefined due to the similar hyperechoic appearance of both the superficial epineurium and the surrounding fat. Generally speaking, nerves are compressible structures and alter their

shape depending on the volume of the anatomical spaces within which they run, as well as on the bulk and conformation of the perineural structures. Across synovial joints, they pass through narrow anatomical passageways – the osteofibrous tunnels – that redirect their course. The floor of these tunnels consists of bone, whereas the roof is made of focal thickenings of the fascia, the so-called "retinacula", which prevent dislocation and traumatic damage of the structures contained in the tunnel during joint activity [43]. In normal states, color and power Doppler US are able to depict blood flow signals from perineural and interfascicular vessels only occasionally and in large nerve trunks.

Careful scanning technique of nerves based on the precise knowledge of their position and analysis of their anatomical relationships with surrounding structures is essential. Systematic scanning on short axis planes is preferred to follow the nerves contiguously throughout the limbs [40]. Once detected, the nerve is kept in the center of the US image in its short axis and then followed proximally and distally shifting the transducer up or down according to its course. With this technique – called the "lift technique" – the examiner is able to explore long segments of a nerve in a few seconds throughout the limbs and extremities. In the event of intrinsic or extrinsic nerve abnormalities, the US examination is more appropriately focused on the area-of-interest using oblique and longitu-

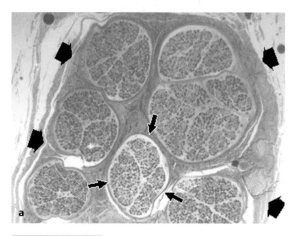 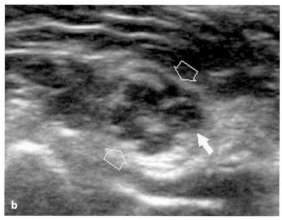

Fig. 3.25 a, b

Nerve echotexture. **a** Histologic slice demonstrates the cross-sectional appearance of a nerve (*large arrows*) composed of many fascicles (*narrow arrows*). **b** Transverse 17-5MHz US image of the ulnar nerve at the arm. The nerve (*empty arrows*) is characterized by a honeycombing appearance made of round hypoechoic areas (*narrow arrow*) in a homogeneous hyperechoic background. The cross-sectional appearance of the hypoechoic rounded areas correlate well with the nerve fascicles seen in **a**

dinal US scanning planes. Although all main nerves can readily be displayed in the extremities due to their superficial position and absence of intervening bone, depiction of the peripheral nervous system is not possible everywhere with US. In fact, most cranial nerves, the nerve roots exiting the dorsal, lumbar and sacral spine, the sympathetic chains and the splanchnic nerves in the abdomen cannot be visualized due to their course being too deep or interposition of bony structures.

3.6 Dermis and hypodermis

The skin represents the external covering of the whole body. Its thickness varies according to different body regions, reaching a maximum thickness at the palm of the hand and the sole of the foot. The skin is divided into two different layers; the external layer is the epidermis, consisting of squamous multistratified epithelium that continues deeply with the dermis, a layer of connective tissue made of cells and collagen fibers lying in an amorphous interstitial substance. The dermis contains blood vessels, nerves, lymphatics, hair follicles and glands.

The hypodermis is found even more deeply and it is made of a tissue rich in collagen fibers and connected to the dermis by fibrous branches. The hypodermis has a complicated structure containing adipose storage inside the subcutaneous adipose tissue. The hypodermal thickness varies according to the examined region and to the patient's personal constitution [14, 23].

Detailed US exploration of the skin is now possible due to high frequency and high resolution transducers. The skin appears as a hyperechoic superficial band of variable thickness and homogeneous structure where it is not possible to differentiate the epidermis from the dermis by ultrasound. The hypodermis, on the contrary, is easily identifiable: it appears as a deep hypoechoic layer, characterized by intersecting curvilinear septa, that correspond to supporting fibrous branches, containing blood vessels well-depicted by color Doppler techniques. The hypodermis is separated from the underlying muscular layer by the superficial aponeurotic fascia, appearing as a double hyperechoic line (Fig. 3.26). Dynamic examination is useful to differentiate adipose from muscular tissue [32].

To diagnose skin disease, the main investigation tends to be clinical examination, eventually supported by histological analysis; US can be useful as a follow-up examination when assessing systemic diseases with skin involvement, such as systemic sclerosis (scleroderma).

Subcutaneous tissue ultrasound examination can also be useful in the diagnosis and staging of some neoplastic lesions such as melanoma, glomus tumours and hemangiomas. It is also used for anthropometric studies in sports medicine to calculate the fat-free mass, which represents an important indicator of physical condition for athletes.

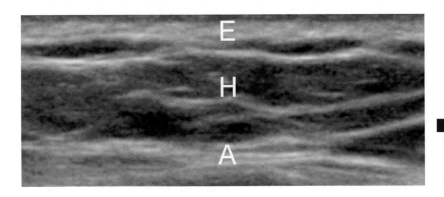

Fig. 3.26

Normal ultrasound appearance of epidermis-dermis (*E*), hypodermis (*H*) and superficial aponeurotic fascia (*A*)

References

1. Grassi W, Cervini C (1998) Ultrasonography in rheumatology: an evolving technique. Ann Rheum Dis 57:268-271
2. Grassi W, Lamanna G, Farina A, Cervini C (1999) Sonographic imaging of normal and osteoarthritic cartilage. Semin Arthritis Rheum 28:398-403
3. McCune WJ, Dedrick DK, Aisen AM, MacGuire A (1990) Sonographic evaluation of osteoarthritic femoral condylar cartilage. Correlation with operative findings. Clin Orthop 254:230-235
4. Martino F, Monetti G (1993) Semeiotica ecografica delle malattie reumatiche. Piccin ed., Padova
5. Sheperd DET, Seedhom BB (1999) Thickness of human articular cartilage in joints of the lower limb. Ann Rheum Dis 58:27-34
6. Aisen AM, McCune WJ, MacGuire A et al (1984) Sonographic evaluation of the cartilage of the knee. Radiology 153:781-784
7. Disler DG, Raymond E, May DA et al (2000) Articular cartilage defects: in vitro evaluation of accuracy and interobserver reliability for detection and grading with US. Radiology 215:846-851
8. Castriota-Scanderbeg A, De Micheli V, Scarale MG et al (1996) Precision of sonographic measurement of articular cartilage: inter- and intraobserver analysis. Skeletal Radiol 25:545-549
9. Backhaus M, Burmester GR, Gerber T et al (2001) Guidelines for musculoskeletal ultrasound in rheumatology. Ann Rheum Dis 60:641-649
10. Grassi W, Tittarelli E, Pirani O et al (1993) Ultrasound examination of metacarpophalangeal joints in rheumatoid arthritis. Scand J Rheumatol 22:243-247
11. Barnett CH, Davies DV, MacConaill MA (1961) Synovial joints. Their structure and mechanics. Longman, London
12. Hlavacek M (1993) The role of synovial fluid filtration by cartilage in lubrification synovial joints. Squeeze film lubrification: homogeneous filtration. J Biomech 26:1151-1160
13. Mc Cutchen CW (1983) Joint lubrification. Bull Hosp Jt dis Orthop Inst 43:118-129
14. Balboni GC et al (1991) Anatomia Umana. Edi-Ermes, Milano
15. Grobbelaar N, Bouffard JA (2000) Sonography of the Knee, a pictorial review. Semin Ultrasound CT MR 21:231-274
16. Bianchi S, Martinoli C, Bianchi-Zamorani M, Valle M (2002) Ultrasound of the joints. Eur. Radiol 12:56-61
17. Wang SC, Chen RK, Cardinal E, Cho KH (1999) Joint sonography. Radiol clin North Am 37:653-668
18. Rindi G, Manni E (1990) Fisiologia umana. Utet, Torino
19. O'Brien M (1992) Functional anatomy ane physiology of tendons. Clin Sports Med 11:505-520
20. Stolinski C (1995) Disposition of collagen fibrils in human tendons. J Anat 186:577-583
21. Ling SC, Chen CF, Wang SC (1990) A study on the vascular supply of the supraspinatus tendon. Surg Radiol Anat 12:161-165
22. Davis WH, Sobel M, Deland J et al (1994) The superior peroneal retinaculum: an anatomic study. Fott Ankle Int 15:271-275
23. Testut L, Latarjet A (1964) Trattato di Anatomia Umana. Utet, Torino
24. Grechenig W, Clement H, Bratschitsch G et al (2002) Ultrasound diagnosis of the Achilles tendon. Orthopade 31:319-325
25. Bruce RK, Hale TL, Gilbert SK (1982) Ultrasonographic evaluation for ruptured Achilles tendon. J Am Pediatr Med Assoc 72:15-17
26. Martinoli C, Derchi LE, Pastorino C et al (1993) Analysis of echotexture of tendons with US. Radiology 186:839-843
27. Jozsa L, Kannus P, Balint JB, Reffy A (1995) Three-dimensional ultrastructure of human tendons. J Anat 142:306-312
28. Dillehay GL et al (1984) The ultrasonographyc characterization of tendons. Invest Radiol 19:338-341
29. Silvestri E, Biggi E, Molfetta L et al (2003) Power Doppler Analysis of tendon vascularization. Int J Tissue React 25:149-158
30. Grassi W, Filippucci E, Farina A, Cervini C (2000) Sonography imaging of the distal phalanx. Semin Arthritis Rheum 29:379-384
31. Bianchi S, Martinoli C, Abdelwahab IF (1999) High-frequency ultrasound examination of the wrist and the hand. Skeletal Radiol 28:121-129
32. Van Holsbeeck M, Introcaso JH (1992) Musculoskeletal Ultrasonography. Radiologic Clinics of North America 5:907-925
33. Narici MV, Maganaris CN, Reeves ND, Capodoglio P (2003) Effect of aging on human muscle and architecture. J Appl Phisiol 95:2229-2234
34. Erickson S (1997) High resolution imaging of the musculoskeletal system. Radiology 205:593-618
35. Balconi G (1993) Apparato locomotore: muscoli e tendini. In: Trattato italiano di ecografia. Poletto Edizioni, Milano
36. Reimens K, Reimens CS, Wagner S et al (1993) Skeletal muscle sonography : a correlative study of echogenicity and morphology. J Ultrasound Med 2:73-77
37. Scott JE (1997) High resolution imaging of the musculoskeletal system. Radiology 205:593-618
38. Bianchi S, Martinoli C, Sureda D, Rizzatto G (2001) Ultrasound of the hand. Eur J Ultrasound 14:29-34
39. Hall MC (1965) The locomotor system: functional anatomy. Thomas, Springfield, Illinois
40. Martinoli C, Bianchi S, Derchi LE (1999) Tendon and nerve sonography. Radiol Clin North Am 37:691-711
41. Beekman R, Visser LH (2004) High-resolution sonography of the peripheral nervous system: a review of the literature. Eur J Neurology 11:305-314
42. Silvestri E, Martinoli C, Derchi LE et al (1995) Echotexture of peripheral nerves: correlation between US and histologic findings and criteria to differentiate tendons. Radiology 197:291-296
43. Martinoli C, Bianchi S, Gandolfo N et al (2000) US of nerve entrapments in osteofibrous tunnels of the upper and lower limbs. Radiographics 20:199-217

Sonographic and power Doppler semeiotics in musculoskeletal disorders

4.1 Cartilage

Sonography has great potential for the non-invasive study of hyaline cartilage, as it can depict microscopic lesions to be demonstrated with a high spatial resolution. The main limit to the sonographic study of articular cartilage is the relatively limited dimensions of acoustic windows available for the visualization of the cartilage surfaces. The most frequent errors in the study of cartilage, especially at knee level, are linked to incorrect examination. The most frequent artifacts come out in suprapatellar panoramic views, as the cartilage profile of the femoral trochlea is not perpendicular to the direction of the US beam. An apparent loss in sharpness of the chondro-synovial margin of the cartilage and an apparent reduction or increase of the cartilage thickness are the main artifacts caused by incorrect technique [2].

Ultrasonography provides rapid and reliable, albeit incomplete, information about the characteristics of articular cartilage, without radiation risk or patient discomfort [3-5].

A wide range of cartilaginous changes can be detected in patients with osteoarthritis and chronic arthritis. These include: *loss of sharpness* of the superficial margin, *loss of transparency* of the cartilaginous layer, *cartilage thinning* and *subchondral bone profile irregularities*.

Osteoarthritis

Cartilage involvement in osteoarthritis ranges from subtle findings to extensive, easily detectable abnormalities [6-8]. Loss of clarity of the cartilage and loss of sharpness of the synovial space-cartilage interface are clearly evident features even in the absence of other US signs of cartilage damage. The integrity of the synovial space-cartilage interface is the main distinguishing feature of healthy subjects, when compared to patients with osteoarthritis (Fig. 4.1). Loss of cartilage transparency could reflect pathological changes such as fibrillation of cartilage and cleft formation.

Blurred and/or irregular margins together with marked cartilage thinning are the most common US findings in advanced osteoarthritis (Fig. 4.2 a, b).

Although standard criteria for assessing US changes in osteoarthritic condylar cartilage are not yet widely accepted, McCune et al. [7] have reported four main abnormalities in patients with knee osteoarthritis that can be regarded as US hallmarks of the disease at different stages. These include loss of cartilage transparency, reduced sharpness of the superficial cartilage margin, increased intensity of the deep cartilage margin and cartilage thinning [8-12].

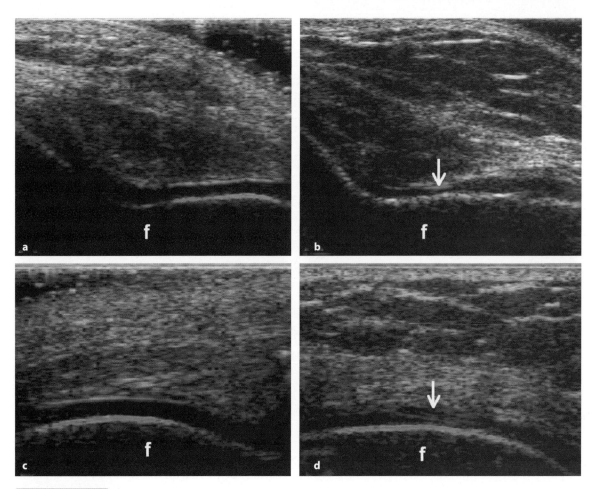

Fig. 4.1 a-d

Osteoarthritis. Transverse (**a**, **b**) and longitudinal (**c**, **d**) supra-patellar US scans of the knee. **a**, **c** Normal cartilage features. **b**, **d** Loss of sharpness of the superficial margin and circumscribed thinning (arrows) of the cartilage layer of the medial femoral condyle (*f*)

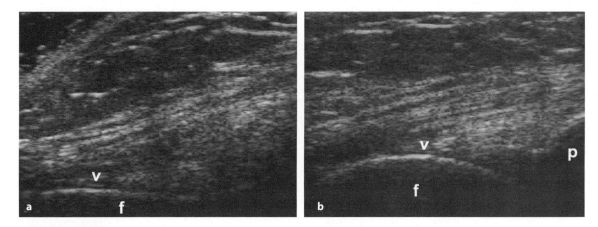

Fig. 4.2 a, b

Osteoarthritis. Transverse (**a**) and longitudinal (**b**) supra-patellar US scans of the knee. Marked diffuse thinning (*arrowheads*) of the cartilage layer of the lateral femoral condyle (*f*). *p* = upper pole of the patella

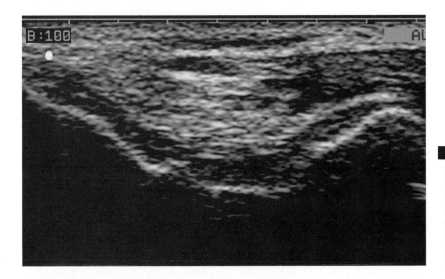

Fig. 4.3

Osteoarthritis. Transverse view of the femoral trochlea in a patient with patello-femoral involvement shows inhomogeneous echogenicity and non-uniform thinning of the articular cartilage, with conspicuously uneven profile of the osteo-chondral interface

Rheumatoid arthritis

US has much to offer in the study of rheumatoid arthritis in spite of the relative lack of scientific reports on the subject. The main drawbacks to research in this field include the current limited availability of very high resolution probes together with the lack of standardized US criteria for cartilage involvement.

In rheumatoid patients, US can visualize pre-erosive changes, particularly at the level of the metacarpophalangeal joint, together with loss of the cartilage layer and irregularities of the subchondral bone (Figs. 4.4, 4.5) [3, 12].

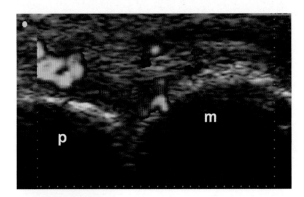

Fig. 4.4

Rheumatoid arthritis. Longitudinal dorsal scan of a metacarpophalangeal joint. Severe cartilage damage involving all the cartilage layer of the metacarpal head. Power Doppler technique shows active pannus invading the subchondral bone. *m* = metacarpal head; *p* = proximal phalanx

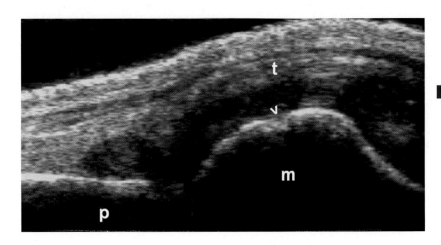

Fig. 4.5

Rheumatoid arthritis. Longitudinal dorsal scan of a metacarpophalangeal joint shows proliferative synovitis with early erosive changes. Complete loss of the cartilage layer of the metacarpal head with initial subchondral involvement (*arrowhead*). *m* = metacarpal head; *p* = proximal phalanx; *t* = extensor tendon

Gout

In patients with long-standing untreated gout, monosodium urate crystal deposition on the surface of the articular cartilage results in hyperechoic enhancement of the superficial margin, which can range from the homogeneous thickening of the synovial space-cartilage interface, to areas of focal deposition (Fig. 4.6 a, b).

Due to the deposition of monosodium urate crystals, reflectivity of the superficial margin is no longer dependant upon the angle of insonation, and a panoramic visualization of the full synovial space-cartilage interface can be easily ascertained, and the amount of crystal deposition estimated. The adherence of monosodium urate crystals to the superficial margin of the articular cartilage can be confirmed by dynamic assessment using active and passive movement of the joint.

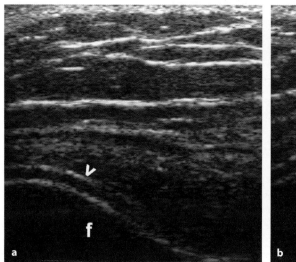 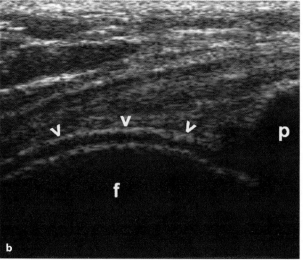

Fig. 4.6 a, b

Chronic gout. Transverse (**a**) and longitudinal (**b**) supra-patellar views of the knee demonstrate diffuse urate crystal deposition (*arrowheads*) on the cartilage surface of the lateral femoral condyle (*f*). *p* = upper pole of the patella

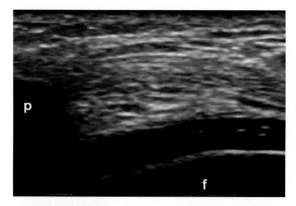

Fig. 4.7

Pyrophosphate arthropathy. Transverse para-patellar view of the knee depicts minimal aggregates of pyrophosphate crystals within the femoral cartilage. *f* = medial femoral condyle; *p* = patella

Pyrophosphate arthropathy

In patients with pyrophosphate arthropathy, crystals are detectable within the substance of the hyaline cartilage (Fig. 4.7) [11-13]. The sparkling reflectivity of pyrophosphate crystals allows for clear depiction of even minimal aggregates within cartilage. Crystal deposition can be focal or diffuse – leading to the development of a 'double contour', which is created by the permeability of the crystal layer, allowing US to penetrate and depict the bone profile beneath.

This is typically seen in the articular cartilage of the femoral condyles and should not be confused with meniscal calcification [9]. One striking feature of this deposition pattern is the apparent geometric location of the crystal layer within the middle portion of

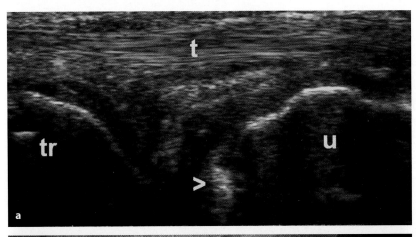

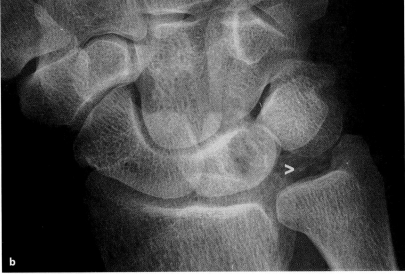

Fig. 4.8 a, b

Pyrophosphate arthropathy. **a** Longitudinal US scan of the ulnar aspect of the wrist. **b** X-ray. Calcification of the triangular ligament of the carpus (*arrowheads*) is evident. *t* = extensor carpi ulnaris tendon; *u* = ulna; *tr* = triquetrum

the articular cartilage, which may help to understand why cartilage is damaged in pyrophosphate arthropathy, leading to secondary degenerative changes.

Calcific deposits in pyrophosphate arthropathy appear as hyperechoic rounded or amorphous shaped areas and their location within the fibrocartilage can be confirmed by dynamic assessment of the joint during real-time scanning. These aggregates can be identified in the menisci of the knee and in the triangular ligament of the wrist. There is close correlation between the appearance of these crystal deposits on X-ray and US (Figs. 4.8 a, b, 4.9 a, b).

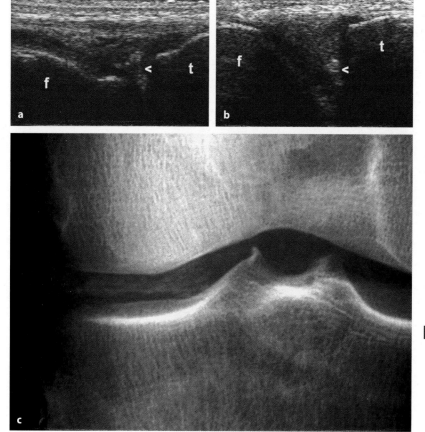

Fig. 4.9 a-c
Pyrophosphate arthropathy of the knee joint. **a, b** US images. **c** X-ray. Lateral (**a**) and medial (**b**) longitudinal US scans demonstrate the presence of calcification of both the menisci (*arrowheads*). *f* = femur; *t* = tibia

4.2 Synovial cavity

Ultrasound is a highly sensitive technique for the detection of even minimal fluid collections and it still represents a particularly useful diagnostic tool to quantify fluid and to monitor its evolution. This latest application is considerably helpful in rheumatological therapy because it constitutes a valid method of evaluation of efficacy. The considerable sensitivity of the identification of synovial fluid collection, the highly detailed anatomical depiction and the real time visualization of tissues make US the ideal imaging technique for interventional guided procedures, such as arthrocentesis. Thanks to US, the aspiration of synovial fluid is even possible even when the joint collection is minimal.

Pathologic conditions that can be assessed within the synovial cavity with US include hydrarthrosis, pneumohydrarthrosis, pyarthrosis, hemarthrosis, lipohemarthrosis, bursitis, tenosynovitis and synovial thickening.

US may occasionally detect the presence of synovial ganglia, joint mice and synovial calcification.

Intracavitary synovial fluid collection

A collection of fluid within the synovial cavity causes the swelling of the involved joint.

In **hydrarthrosis**, US shows fluid collection within the cavity, which has an anechoic appearance with dorsal acoustic enhancement (Fig. 4.10 a, b).

The amount of fluid within the joint is directly proportional to the severity of the synovial inflammation and to the capability of the capsular wall to expand. In some cases the anechoic appearance of the fluid collection can be inhomogeneous because of the presence of dot-like echoes scattered within the collection itself [14-16]. This more complicated appearance of the collection may depend on the presence of a fibrinous component within the inflammatory exudate, which can be particularly abundant in relapsing collections and can be

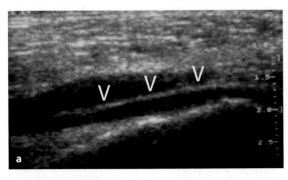 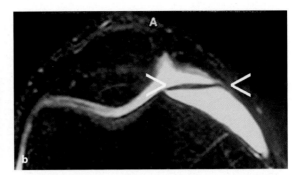

Fig. 4.10 a, b

a US scan of medial paracondylar recess. Anechoic reactive fluid collection containing a thin septum (physiological medio-patellar plica, *arrowheads*). **b** Axial fat suppression sequence magnetic resonance (MR) scan confirms the presence of mediopatellar plica (*arrowheads*), which appear as low signal bundle within the hyperintense articular fluid collection

visualized as arranged echogenic and inhomogeneous clusters, with a scirrhous conformation.

Pyarthrosis occurs in bacterial arthritis, which is usually rare in patients with normal immune systems, while it is common in children, in immunosuppressed patients, in diabetics and in patients on dialysis. In acute infections with joint fluid collection, it is necessary to sample the fluid in order to prescribe the most appropriate antibiotic therapy. In chronic infections the fluid collection is usually poor and it is often associated with considerable synovial thickening. In infections the fluid is usually hypoechoic, but it may appear hyperechoic in more superficial joints. In such cases, the synovial hyperemia can be well-depicted with the use of Doppler techniques as a complement to gray scale US [17, 18]. However, it should be kept in mind that synovial hyperemia in bacterial arthritis is not a mandatory finding, because it depends on the patient's age, on the duration of the infection and on the immune status. Therefore, since there is no certainty in differentiating septic from aseptic inflammation and it is more suitable to perform a biopsy when clinical suspicion is high.

Hemarthrosis exhibit a peculiar US pattern that changes with time similar to hematoma. Hemorrhagic fluid collections are in fact homogeneously echogenic within the first two to three days from onset, due to the presence of a corpuscular content. After the third day, the hemarthrosis shows a progressive reduction in echogenicity due to lytic enzyme release. Eventually, US shows echogenic branches, corresponding to fibrinous clots, crossing the anechoic-appearing zone [14, 15].

Occasionally, the post-arthrocentesis follow-up examination demonstrates the presence of **pneumohydrarthrosis**. The presence of gas in the joint cavity produces a highly reflective mist within the anechoic fluid collection, forming an air-fluid level that changes together with the patient's position. When assessing hydrarthrosis and pneumohydrarthrosis, color and power Doppler techniques do not demonstrate significant vascular changes [3, 17, 18].

Lipohemarthrosis is easily identified by means of US and it appears as a dual-phase collection, showing a fluid-fluid level. The overlying echogenic fraction corresponds to the lipid content, while the underlying fraction is hemorrhagic. When lipohemarthrosis is found in a post-traumatic limb, the presence of a joint fracture can be suspected.

Synovial thickening

Hypertrophic or hyperplasic synovial thickening is a condition found in several long-standing inflammatory arthropathies and it can be the cause of bone and cartilage erosion in the joint.

US nowadays can identify inflammatory synovial thickening more accurately than clinical examination, especially when small joints such as the metacarpophalangeal and interphalangeal joints are affected, commonly observed in chronic polyarthropathies. Synovial thickening is characterized by heterogeneous echotexture varying from hypoechoic to hyperechoic, depending on the amount of water contained in the synovial tissue

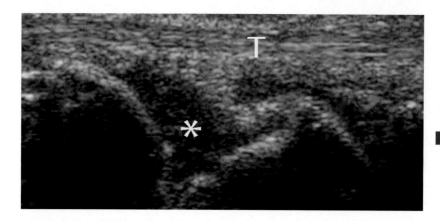

Fig. 4.11

Longitudinal sonogram of wrist, dorsal side in a patient affected by rheumatoid arthritis. Synovial proliferation appears hypoechoic (*). *T* = extensor tendons

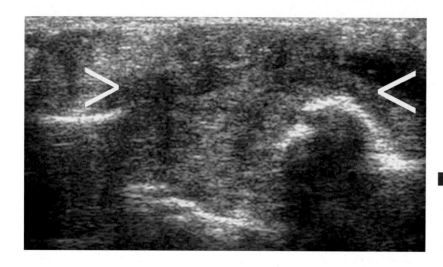

Fig. 4.12

Longitudinal sonogram of wrist, dorsal side. Patient affected by rheumatoid arthritis. In this case, synovial proliferation (*arrowheads*) has a hyperechoic appearance

(Figs. 4.11, 4.12). In larger joints, such as the knee, the synovial thickening appears as a succession of irregularly proliferating branches, mildly echoic, jutting out from the synovia into the articular cavity; the assessment of synovial pannus is considerably easier when associated with a fluid collection because it works as a contrast agent [1, 14-16] (Fig. 4.13).

In pigmented villonodular synovitis, the synovial hypertrophy is usually overabundant, made of thick fusiform villi and gross nodules, with a winding outline surrounded by abundant fluid collection. A similar appearance can be observed in joints affected by relapsing hemarthrosis in hemophilic arthropathies. The continual presence of hemorragic effusion irritates the synovial membrane and determines the formation of pannus that starts as a simple thickening and then turns into villous hypertrophy. The sonographer should always

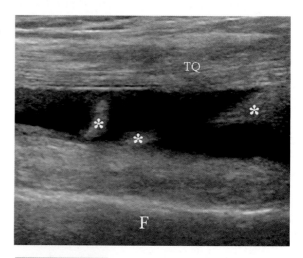

Fig. 4.13

Longitudinal US scan of supra-patellar recess showing large amount of anechoic fluid collection with hyperechoic synovial proliferation (*). *TQ* = quadricipital tendon; *F* = femur

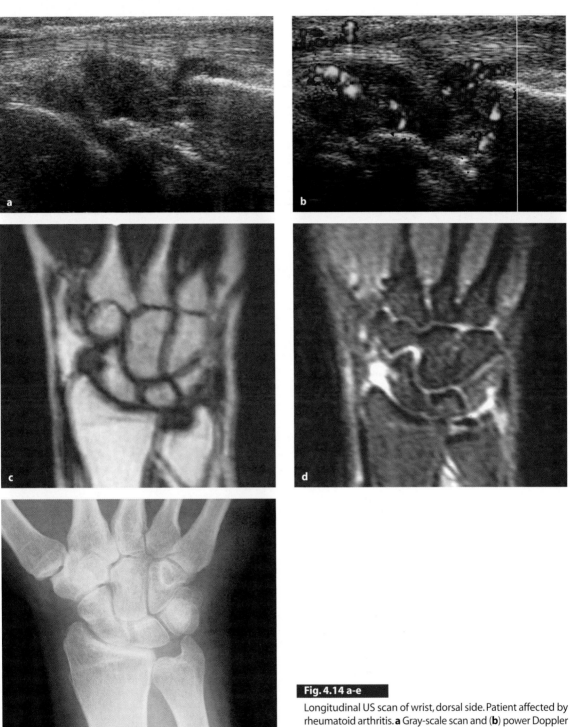

Fig. 4.14 a-e

Longitudinal US scan of wrist, dorsal side. Patient affected by rheumatoid arthritis. **a** Gray-scale scan and (**b**) power Doppler scan. The use of power Doppler allows the amount of synovial proliferation to be assessed more than MR without contrast (spin echo T1 (SET1), short T1 inversion recovery (STIR)) (**c, d**) or a plain film (**e**)

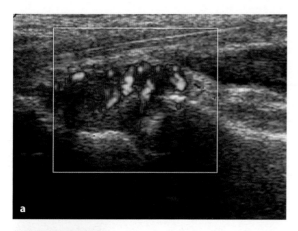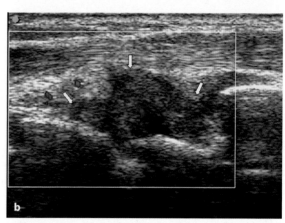

Fig. 4.15 a, b

Patient with rheumatoid arthritis. **a** The power Doppler scan shows a high degree of hyperperfusion, an expression of hyperactive pannus. **b** Follow-up during therapy. A significant reduction in flow signal is shown within the pannus (*arrows*)

keep in mind that synovial hypertrophy is a non-specific finding and that the differentiation between a non-specific synovitis and a synovial tumor can be very tricky (hemangioma, synovial sarcoma) [14-16]. A fibrinous exudate can make it difficult to detect the thickened synovial membrane contour, especially when it is abundant, because it may simulate the US pattern of synovial hyperplasia. In these cases, when fluid and hypertrophic synovia cannot be differentiated it is possible to use dynamic and compressive maneuvers. Such a technique allows the fluid to be "squeezed out" from the hypertrophic synovial wall and the differentiation of the two articular contents [1, 14, 16].

When doubt persists with gray-scale US, power and color Doppler techniques can be applied to differentiate the fluid from the proliferating tissue, with the presence or absence of vascular signals [17-20] (Fig. 4.14 a-e).

The role of Doppler techniques for the assessment of synovial vascularization in rheumatoid arthritis is very important. In rheumatoid arthritis, the formation of pannus is a crucial event in the pathogenesis of articular degeneration. Neoangiogenesis is an important pathological element in rheumatoid synovitis [21, 22]. Since hypervascu-

larization is proportional to the degree of inflammation of the synovial pannus, it is fundamental to study and quantify the vascular signals in order to evaluate the aggressiveness of the pannus itself. Power Doppler is able to assess the increased vascularization involving synovial hyperplasic tissue and consequently to give information regarding the activity of the synovial pannus [1, 18-20] (Fig. 4.15 a, b). Despite attempts at semiquantitative or quantitative evaluation of the vascularization by means of dedicated software, the technique is limited by the poor reproducibility.

Nevertheless, the recent availability of power Doppler techniques in association with the use of contrast agents (Contrast-enhanced Power Doppler – CePD) has allowed a more detailed analysis of the synovial vascularization. It should be considered that the information derived from power Doppler and CePD refer exclusively to the macrovasculature of synovial pannus. Such limits have now been overcome by the introduction of new generation contrast agents (SonoVue) that allow quantitative analysis of the synovial microvascularization to be performed by means of gray-scale US (Contrast-enhanced US – CeUS) [23-25] (Fig. 4.16 a-c).

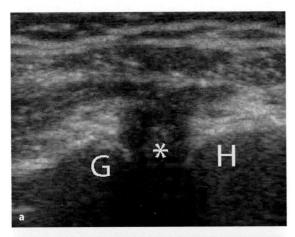

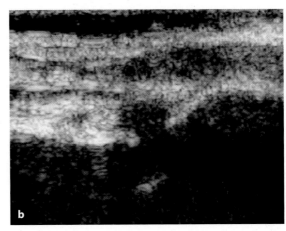

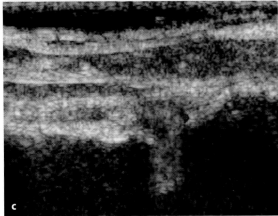

Fig. 4.16 a-c

Patient with rheumatoid arthritis. **a** Shoulder, posterior scan. Expansion of posterior capsular recess with inhomogeneous hypoechoic synovial proliferation (*). **b**, **c** Images taken before (**b**), and after (**c**), injection of contrast agent (Ce-US). These scans show a significant hyperemia of synovial proliferation. The hyperechoic appearance is due to the contrasting microbubbles. G = posterior margin of humeral glenoid process; H = posterior aspect of humeral head

Bursitis

Bursae are anatomical entities located near joints (non-communicating bursae) or in direct communication with the joint cavity (communicating bursae). The main function of non-communicating bursae, located at the insertional areas of the anchor tendons of several joints, is to reduce the friction between tendon and bone. Communicating bursae, on the other hand, when an abundant intra-articular fluid collection occurs, function by reducing the joint cavity pressure, by expanding and being filled with the fluid coming from the cavity.

Bursitis represents the most common bursal pathology and US is the first choice diagnostic technique.

Non-communicating bursitis

a. **Acute traumatic bursitis:** affecting several synovial bursae, the bursal expansion follows direct impact or chronic frictional microtrauma. The most commonly involved bursae are the sub-

acromial-deltoid bursa, the pre-patellar and deep infra-patellar bursa, the retro-calcaneal and superficialis bursa of the Achilles tendon and the trochanteric bursa. In acute forms, an increase in anechoic fluid within the bursa is observed (a comparison with the controlateral limb may be useful), while the synovial wall keeps its original thickness (Fig. 4.17 a, b). In chronic forms, the fluid often appears hypoechoic and contains hyperechoic spots consistent with microcalcification, and the bursal walls are thickened [26] (Fig. 4.18 a, b).

b. **Hemorrhagic bursitis:** usually following a violent sporting trauma on artificial surfaces and mainly affect the hands and knees. The hemorrhagic effusion may organize and form adhesions or calcifications. Clots and fibrin, appearing as irregular hyperechoic masses, are easily distinguished from synovial hypertrophy because of their mobility and the absence of vascular signal on power or color Doppler analysis.

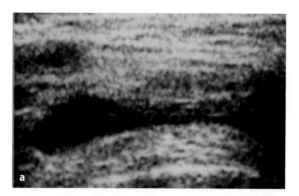

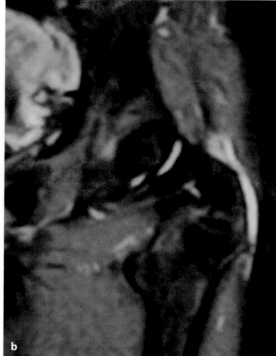

Fig. 4.17 a, b

a Longitudinal scan of the lateral aspect of the left hip. Inflammatory distension of trochanteric bursa with hypoechoic fluid inside. **b** MR scan of the same patient (coronal, fat suppression technique)

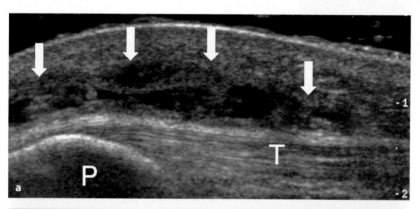

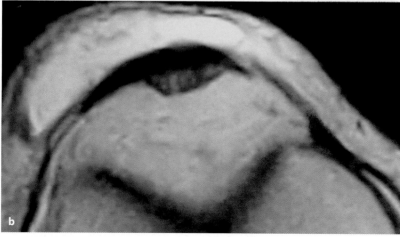

Fig. 4.18 a, b

a Anterior compartment of knee, longitudinal scan. Post-traumatic distension of pre-patellar bursa (*arrows*) with a small amount of fluid and thin echoic septa. *P* = patella; *T* = patellar tendon. **b** MR scan of the same patient (axial, turbo spin echo (TSE) T2)

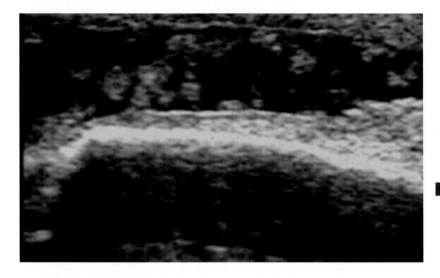

Fig. 4.19

Patient with gout, olecranon bursitis. The bursa is expanded by a small amount of synovial fluid with some hyperechoic synovial proliferation

c. **Chemical bursitis:** often associated with metabolic disease, inflammatory and degenerative processes. The most common cause is the monosodium urate crystals deposition in gout.

d. **Septic bursitis:** difficult to differentiate from chronic inflammatory bursitis, but it is characterized by intrabursal hyperechoic diffuse areas, corresponding to thickened synovial membrane (Fig. 4.19). The presence of gas within the bursa may be consistent with septic bursitis, but the final diagnosis can be obtained by performing a color or power Doppler examination that allows the detection of vascular signals within the soft tissues, indicating a inflammatory hyperemia, or, even better, by sampling the bursal fluid [1, 18-20].

Communicating bursitis

Communicating synovial bursae develop during adolescence and are characterized by the presence of a tract that connects them to the nearby joint. Their function is to reduce intra-articular pressure in order to avoid the onset of joint complications. The most common communicating bursitis is the medial gastrocnemius and semimembranosus tendon bursitis, with a particularly high incidence in rheumatoid arthritis compared with other rheumatic disorders such as Reiter's syndrome, villonodular arthrosynovitis, Sjogren's syndrome, ankylosing spondylitis, psoriatic arthritis, gonococcal arthritis and gout [1, 16] (Fig. 4.20 a, b). In long standing fluid collections, the progressive filling of the bursa leads to the formation of a cyst (Baker's

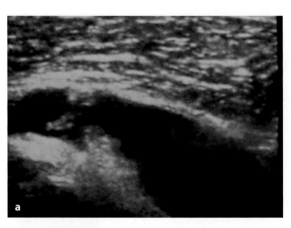

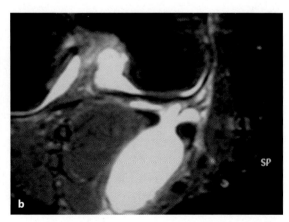

Fig. 4.20 a, b

a Transverse US scan of popliteal fossa in a patient affected by gonarthrosis. Baker's cyst is shown. **b** MR scan of the same patient (axial view, fat suppression technique)

cyst), which can be easily palpated on clinical examination when it reaches considerable dimensions (gigantic cysts) and can be completely visible thanks to panoramic imaging (extended field of view (EFV)) (Fig. 4.21).

The US appearance of a Baker's cyst is that of a hypo-anechoic pear-shaped cavity, with a well-defined outline, presenting with posterior acoustic enhancement. Communication with the superior aspect of the postero-medial edge of the articular cavity can often be detected at the medial femoral condyle. Echoes within the cyst confirm the presence of debris and clots that, especially when abundant, make the US detection of small popliteal cysts difficult [1, 14-16] (Fig. 4.22).

The dimension of a Baker's cyst at follow-up can correlate with the clinical progression of arthritis and the efficacy of medical therapy and, in selected cases, US may be used as a guide for the aspiration and injection of the cyst [1, 14] (Fig. 4.23 a, b).

When swelling is appreciated in the popliteal fossa, it is necessary to perform an US to differentiate a Baker's cyst from vascular (popliteal artery aneurysms, venous thrombosis), or muscular (different degrees of injuries involving the popliteal fossa muscles) pathologies. In chronic inflammatory arthropathies, hypertrophic synovial tissue is observed, with a particularly abundant and irregular appearance in rheumatoid arthritis. In this case the bursa may grow considerably, surrounding the tendon of the medial gastrocnemius muscle (Fig. 4.24).

Sometimes a gigantic cyst may end up rupturing leading to inflammation of the surrounding adipose tissue and of the myofascial components, so that it clinically simulates a thrombophlebitis (pseudo-thrombophlebitic syndrome). A fresh rupture of a gigantic cyst can be detected by US by hazy appear-

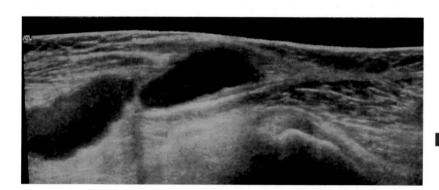

Fig. 4.21

Giant popliteal cyst. This EFV longitudinal scan shows a panoramic view of the multiloculate cyst

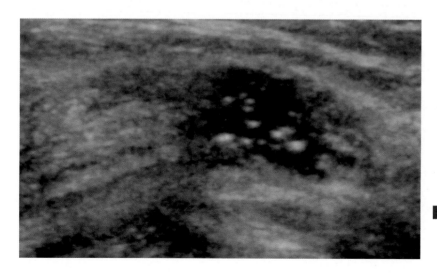

Fig. 4.22

Small popliteal cyst with fluid content and hyperechoic spots, caused by small clots and debris

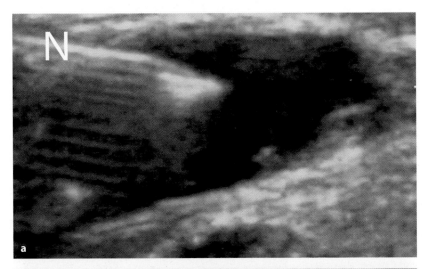

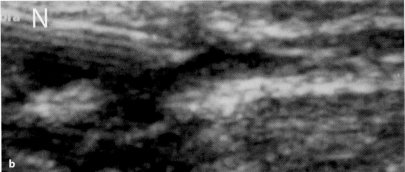

Fig. 4.23 a, b

Popliteal cyst before (**a**) and after (**b**) US-guided aspiration. N = needle. The reverberation artifact is clearly shown

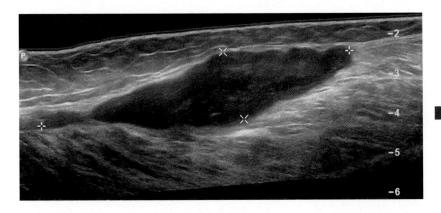

Fig. 4.24

Patient affected with rheumatoid arthritis. The EFV scan shows the whole extent of a giant popliteal cyst that courses toward the proximal third of the leg and has hemorragic content

ance of the cyst's fundus, with an associated free fluid collection located superficially and distally from the cyst itself. When doubt persists, gray-scale US and color or power Doppler techniques play a fundamental role in the differential diagnosis.

In normal circunstances the subacromion-deltoid bursa of the shoulder does not communicate with the joint cavity, whilst in cases of complete rupture of the rotator cuff, direct connection between the two cavities is observed [27] (Fig. 4.25 a, b).

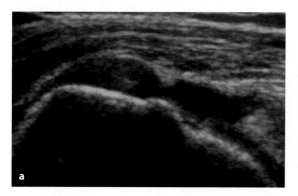

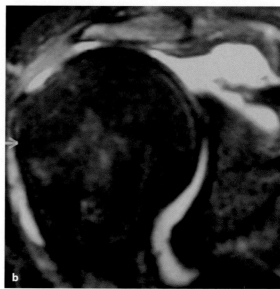

Fig. 4.25 a, b

Complete rupture of rotator cuff. **a** US scan shows a complete tear of supraspinatus tendon. **b** In this case, MR shows the expansion of the articular capsule and of the subacromion-deltoid bursa (fat suppression technique)

Synovial ganglia

Synovial ganglia are mostly found in the upper limb, particularly at the wrist and hand. The most common location is the carpal dorsum. In this case the cyst usually arises from the scapho-lunate joint because of mucoid degeneration phenomena of the tissues due to repeated microtrauma. US allows the ganglion to be visualized as a typical hypo-anechoic nodule, with irregular margins, presenting internal thin hyperechoic septa and a slender peduncle that connects it to the scapho-lunate joint (Fig. 4.26 a, b). The application of dynamic maneuvers to the standard ultrasound examination can be particularly useful for the detection of the connecting peduncle and for better assessment of the cyst's relationships with the surrounding tissues [28-32].

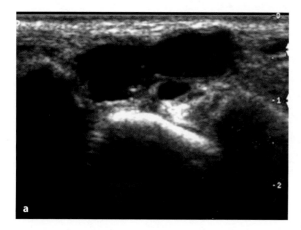

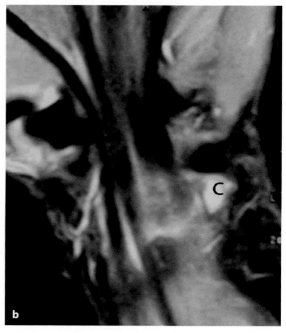

Fig. 4.26 a, b

a Ganglion cyst of radiocarpal joint. Note the polycystic shape with small echogenic septa inside. **b** MR scan in the same patient (coronal scan, fat suppression tecnique). The cyst is homogeneous and hyperintense (*C*)

Endoarticular loose bodies

These can be found in all joints but mostly the knee, where they can be easily detected when located in the suprapatellar recess. Loose bodies occur in several pathologies such as osteochondritis dissecans, osteochondral fractures, osteonecrosis, osteoarthritis, synovial osteochondromatosis. Since they have a highly calcified content, they appear on US as hyperechoic curvilinear bodies, with posterior acoustic shadowing, and are mobile, depending on the patient's position. The mobility of a loose body can be demonstrated, in dubious cases, by dynamic passive maneuvers that also help differentiate it from gross osteophytes. When a loose body contains osteochondral tissue, the cartilaginous covering (hypoechoic) can be differentiated from the bony component [33] (Fig. 4.27 a-c).

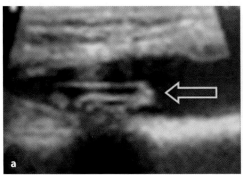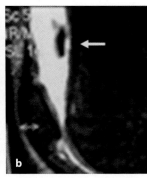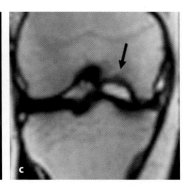

Fig. 4.27 a-c

Loose endoarticular osteochondral body in the supra-patellar recess. **a** The US scan shows a double-layered loose body (*empty white arrow*) due to its dual composition (cartilage and bone). The MR scan (fat suppression technique) (**b**) confirms the presence of the loose body in the supra-patellar recess (*white arrow*) and shows the osteochondral detachment location (*black arrow*) on the femoral condyle (TSE T2, **c**)

Synovial calcifications

Synovial calcification appears on US as a hyperechoic "plate-like" area with posterior acoustic shadowing. The calcified plates, following the synovial membrane outline, have a linear or coarsely wavy appearance and do not move, even when compression is applied with the transducer. This sonographic pattern is typical of synovial osteochondromatosis, but can also be found, less frequently, in chondrocalcinosis and in scleroderma; the calcification process may involve both the synovial membrane of joints and that of mucosal bursae and of tenosynovial sheaths [13, 34].

4.3 Tendons and ligaments

Nowadays, US is the imaging tool of first choice for the study of tendons. Compared to other imaging techniques, such as MR, US allows *static evaluation*, with a highly detailed representation of the intrinsic anatomic structure of tendons and a *dynamic evaluation*, which is an extremely important element for an accurate diagnosis. Tendons are divided, from an anatomic and functional point of view, into two types: 1) *supporting tendons* and 2) *sliding tendons*. This distinction is extremely important in order to understand the most common pathological conditions, both rheumatological and traumatic. In inflammatory tendinopathies all the layers of the tendons are involved (*paratenonitis*), while the tendon's parenchyma (collagen fibers, proteoglycans) is usually only affected in degenerative conditions (*tendinosis*), where the two pathologic conditions often coexist [35].

Moreover, paratenonitis can be distinguished in *tenosynovitis* and *peritendinitis*, according to the specific involvement of sliding tendons or supporting tendons.

Inflammatory and degenerative involvement of the osteo-tendinous junction is called *enthesopathy* and is very common in seronegative spondyloarthritis, but it can also be the expression of a microcristalline arthropathy, or the result of chronic functional overuse of the osteotendinous junction.

Tendon tears and *dislocations* usually follow mechanical overload which exceeds the resistance threshold of the system, the latter being the final expression of a potential instability of sliding tendons lying in critical areas.

Tendon cysts represent quite a common condition, frequently found in the hand and causing painful swelling [36-40].

Tenosynovitis

Tenosynovitis is an inflammatory process affecting the tenosynovial sheath. Tenosynovitis can be classified as *acute*, *subacute* or *chronic*, while from a pathologic point of view they are distinguished in *exudative*, *proliferative* and *mixed* forms. Even though the clinical diagnosis of tenosynovitis may seem easy, the distinction between the different pathologic forms can instead be difficult without US examination, which allows an easy and quick diagnosis to be made.

A peculiar form of tenosynovitis is the *chronic stenosing tenosynovitis*, affecting biomechanically critical anatomic regions. [41-43].

An ***exudative tenosynovitis*** can be easily diagnosed by means of US. In this case, an increase of fluid is seen within the tenosynovial sheath appearing as an anechoic halo surrounding the tendon in axial views, and lying along the tendon course in longitudinal views, frequently with a fusiform appearance (Fig.4.28 a, b).

Sometimes increased echogenicity of the tenosynovial fluid collection may be observed, due to the presence of clusters of leucocytes, fibrin, cholesterol, uric acid, calcium pyrophosphate or hydroxyapatite crystals. This hyperechoic appearance may create doubts about the diagnosis of exudative tenosynovitis and, in such cases, compression made with the transducer may help to confirm the liquid nature of the finding. Power Doppler analysis gives no evidence of vascular signal, therefore it can be used to complement the information obtained with gray-scale US [1, 15, 36, 44]. It should be pointed out that in some anatomical locations, the tenosynovial sheath may be in communication with the joint cavity. For example, the tenosynovial sheaths of the flexor hallucis longus tendon at the ankle and the long head of biceps tendon at the shoulder are in communication with the tibio-talar and gleno-humeral joint. In these cases, when the sheath is expand-

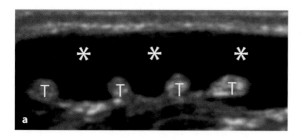

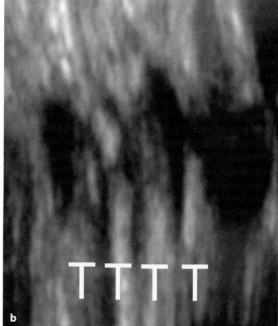

Fig. 4.28 a, b

a Transverse scan, dorsum of wrist (compound imaging). Distension with anechoic fluid (*) of the sheath of the 4th extensor's compartment. **b** MPR reconstruction on a coronal plane.
T = extensors

ed with fluid the presence of a joint fluid collection must be considered.

In *proliferative tenosynovitis* hypertrophic proliferation of the synovial tissue is observed, showing various degrees of echogenicity (Fig. 4.29).

Dynamic ultrasound examination and compression of the transducer performed by the operator are helpful to assess the solid nature of the finding. In these cases the power Doppler analysis is very useful to confirm the diagnosis by detecting vascular signals within a thickened tenosynovial sheath (Fig. 4.30). The degree of vascularization is strictly related to the severity of the inflammation and to the "activity" of the synovial proliferation [15, 18, 21, 36]. These forms of tenosynovitis are often an extra-articular expression of some rheumatic diseases such as rheumatoid arthritis.

Mixed tenosynovitis is the most common form of tenosynovitis. It is characterized by the simultaneous presence of both synovial fluid and proliferative thickening of the synovial membrane within the sheath. The US pattern shows several echoic spots of synovial tissue jutting from the sheath expanded by anechoic fluid (Fig. 4.31).

In order to differentiate fluid from the proliferating tissue it is very useful to apply compres-

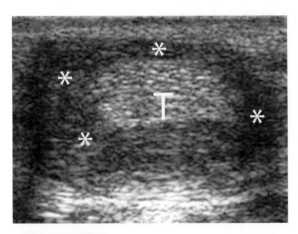

Fig. 4.29

Transverse scan, finger flexor tendons. Expansion of the tendon sheath with hyperechoic synovial proliferation (*) is shown

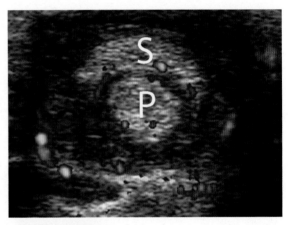

Fig. 4.30

Transverse power Doppler scan, finger flexor tendons. Proliferative tenosinovitis with diffuse hypervascularization is shown. S = flexor superficialis tendon; P = flexor profundus tendon

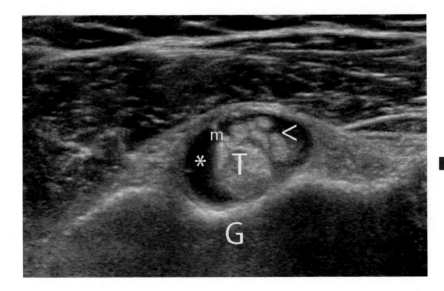

Fig. 4.31

Long head of biceps tendon of the shoulder, transverse scan. Fluid expansion (*) of the synovial sheath with synovial proliferation (*arrowheads*) is shown (mixed tenosynovitis). m = mesotenonium; G = intertubercular groove; T = tendon

sion with the transducer. In dubious cases the two components can also be distinguished with power Doppler, because vascular signals exclusively occur within the solid tissue.

In all cases where inflammatory involvement of the tenosynovial sheath is observed, US evaluation of the tendon's morphology and intrinsic structure should be performed. Tendon presenting with an alteration of their echotexture express concomitant pathologic involvement of its parenchyma [15, 44] (Fig. 4.32).

Chronic stenosing tenosynovitis occurs in peculiar anatomical regions, where the tendons run through fibro-osseous canals. The most common US pattern is that of a mixed tenosynovitis, accompanied by thickening of the corresponding retinaculum and consequent stenosis of the canal. From a functional point of view, the dynamic US examination may demonstrate a defective sliding of the tendon within the sheath. Notta-Nelaton's disease, also known as "trigger finger", and De Quervain's disease are the most common forms of chronic stenosing tenosynovitis [1, 45, 46] (Fig. 4.33).

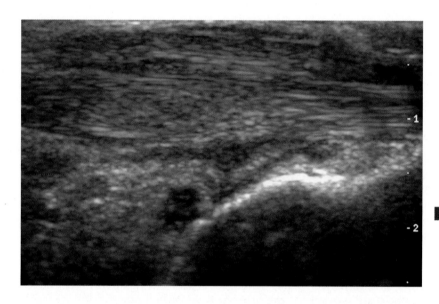

Fig. 4.32

Ankle, longitudinal scan. Tendinosis and inflammatory expansion of the sheath. Thickening of fibular tendons and inhomogeneous echotexture is shown

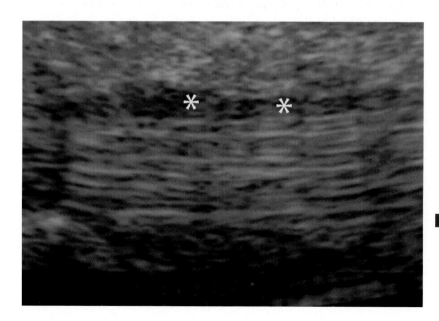

Fig. 4.33

Chronic stenosing tenosynovitis of 1st compartment of extensors (abductor pollicis longus and extensor pollicis brevis). Enlargement (*) of tenosynovial sheath (20 MHz transducer)

Peritendinitis

The term peritendinitis refers to inflammation of the paratenon of anchor tendons, especially involving the highly vascular loose areolar connective tissue that is found between epitenon and peritenon. In practice, peritendinitis of anchor tendons corresponds to tenosynovitis of sliding tendons, for they both represent a paratenonitis.

Peritendinitis often affects tendons of the lower limbs, particularly the patellar and Achilles tendons. Like tenosynovitis, peritendinitis can be classified as *acute*, *subacute* or *chronic*. The most common cause of peritendinitis is repeated microtrauma [35]. US highlights the inflammatory edema, a hypoechoic thickening of the peritendinous wrapping layers (Fig. 4.34) with a hypoechoic ring-like appearance in short axis views. In the classic pattern of peritendinitis, the fibrillar tendon echotexture does not appear altered; it is altered instead in mixed forms where peritendinitis and tendinosis coexist.

The information obtained with gray-scale US can be usefully integrated with an accurate color and power Doppler analysis that can add further information regarding the presence of peritendinous inflammation and hyperemia. It should also be mentioned that in standard conditions the vascularization of tendons is very poor with low speed flow, invisible on Doppler analysis. When hyperemia is detected, a typical hypervascular pattern is observed; this is characterized by several signal spots and typically located in the peritendinous area [47, 48] (Fig. 4.35).

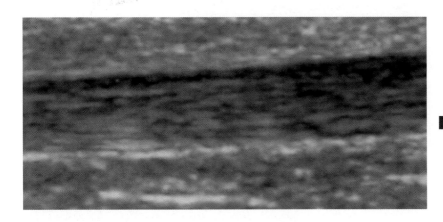

Fig. 4.34

Peritendinitis of the Achilles tendon. Longitudinal scan, compound imaging. Thin peritendinous layer of hypoechoic fluid with normal thickness of tendon is shown

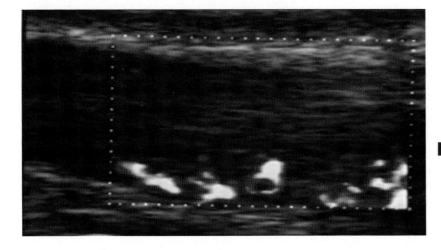

Fig. 4.35

Peritendinitis of the Achilles tendon. The power Doppler scan shows some peritendineal vascular signals, expression of hyperemia and inflammation of tendon sheath

Tendinosis

Tendinosis is a degenerative pathology affecting both anchor and sliding tendons, presenting with mild pain or with no symptoms at all. Consequently, US plays a fundamental role in diagnosis, because the patient's history and clinical examination alone cannot accurately implicate the involved tendon. From a histopathologic point of view, fibroblasts are activated with the production of high molecular weight collagen and proteogly-cans, causing diffuse edema. Necrosis and fibrinous exudation occur with a probable consequent fibrocartilaginous metaplasia and calcium deposition. US is able to detect tendon alteration in early phases. The earliest US sign of tendinosis, in long axis views, is disarray of tendon echotexture and its fusiform thickening corresponding, in short axis views, to the rounded appearance with loss of the typical ventral concavity. In early US patterns of tendinosis, fragmentation of the fibrillar echotexture is observed [49] (Fig. 4.36).

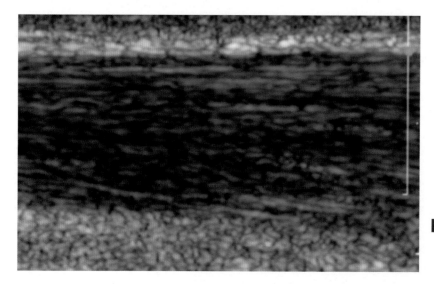

Fig. 4.36

Low grade tendinosis. The characteristic fragmentation of the fibrillar echotexture is shown

In later phases, focal hypoechoic areas, related to mucoid degeneration can be observed (Fig.4.37). Collagen fibers show a lack of organization; several hyperechoic spots can be detected, suggesting the presence of micro and macro-calcification. The largest hyperechoic spots show posterior acoustic shadowing, representing areas of calcific metaplasia within the tendon [50] (Fig. 4.38).

Further assessment of intratendinous hypoechoic focal areas using color or power Doppler techniques can be useful to detect vascular signals within the degenerative spots, a finding suggestive of the presence of angiogenesis, with a potential consequent substitution of the degenerate area. The absence of vascular signals within the degenerate areas of the tendon suggests necrotic evolution of the degenerative focus. It

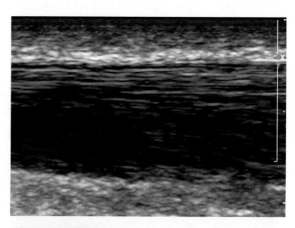

Fig. 4.37

Tendinosis of Achilles tendon. The tendon is thickened and inhomogeneous with an extensive hypoechoic area (mucoid intratendinous degeneration)

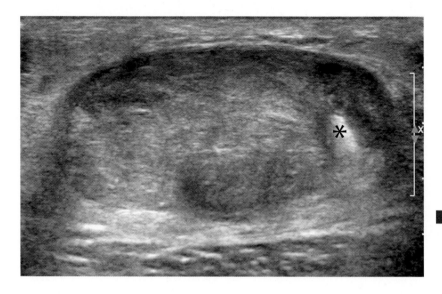

Fig. 4.38

Transverse scan of Achilles tendinosis. The tendon is thickened and inhomogeneous with a small focus of calcification (*)

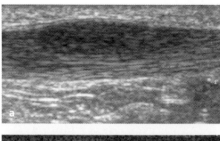

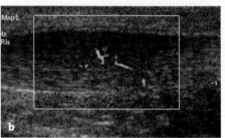

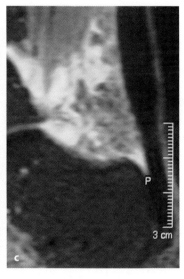

Fig. 4.39 a-c

a Longitudinal scan of Achilles tendinosis. The tendon is thickened, inhomogeneous and devoid of its characteristic fibrillar echotexture. **b** The power Doppler scan shows some intratendinous vascular signals. **c** MR scan of the same patient (fat suppression technique). Diffuse hyperintensity of Kager's triangle caused by inflammation of the adipose tissue

should be mentioned that in clinical practice it is common to find cases in which an overlap between degenerative (tendinosis) and inflammatory (paratenonitis) tendon conditions occurs, and in these cases the complex color and power Doppler images can be integrated with gray-scale US to give a more precise assessment [47] (Fig. 4.39 a-c).

It should also be considered that some anatomical regions present peculiar biomechanical characteristics that promote the onset of tendinosis.

For instance, the presence of a prominent postero-superior calcaneal tubercle (Haglund's disease) may cause friction with the pre-insertional portion of the Achilles tendon. In these cases, ultrasound shows the presence of inflammatory and degenerative tendon involvement, especially located at the pre-insertional portion, which appears thickened and inhomogeneous and is often associated with a precalcaneal and retrocalcaneal bursitis [51] (Fig. 4.40 a, b).

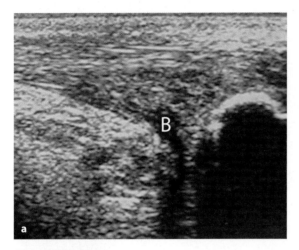
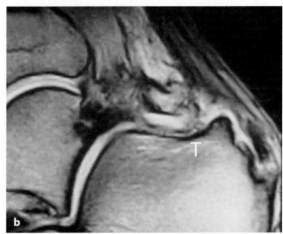

Fig. 4.40 a, b

Haglund disease. **a** Longitudinal scan. The pre-insertional segment of Achilles tendon appears inhomogeneous and thickened, with inflammation of the retro-calcaneal bursa (B). **b** MR scan of the same patient (gradient echo (GE) T2W sequence). The US diagnosis is confirmed by the presence of a prominent postero-superior calcaneal tubercle. *T* = tubercle

Enthesopathy

Enthesopathy, also known as insertional tendinopathy, is an inflammatory-degenerative pathology involving the osteo-tendinous junction, usually caused by functional overload. It typically affects anchor tendons submitted to continual and intense mechanical stress. The affected anatomical region, therefore, varies according to the athletic task, resulting in the onset of typical pathologies associated with specific sports, such as tennis elbow and jumper's knee.

In standard conditions the enthesis consists of intertwined tendon fibers and fibrocartilage, with slow flowing vessels that cannot be visualized on Doppler analysis. In enthesopathies, the earliest pathologic finding is local hyperemia and angiogenesis; with Doppler techniques the increase of vascular signals can be identified early, when the matrix of tendons is not yet altered. US is a highly sensitive technique for identifying and quantifying the tendon insertional thickening, the hypoechoic pattern and the inhomogeneous echotexture. Insertional calcification and hypoechoic focal areas, corresponding to myxoid degeneration within the tendon, may be observed [52] (Fig. 4.41).

An inflammatory reaction of the adjacent serous bursa and the presence of erosions and of an irregular cortical bone outline at the insertion are often associated. On US, erosions appear as interruptions of the hyperechoic cortical bone outline. In advanced cases, an MR examination should be per-

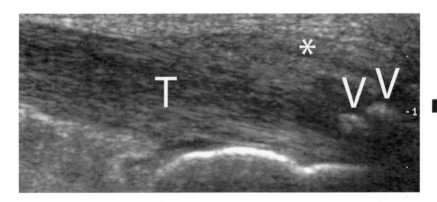

Fig. 4.41

Longitudinal scan of Achilles tendon (*T*) enthesopathy. Diffuse disarray of the fibrillar echotexture, calcifications (*arrowheads*) and thickening of peri-calcaneal soft tissues (*)

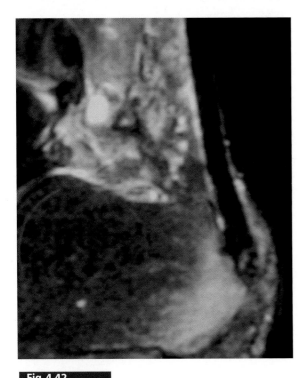

Fig. 4.42

MR of the ankle, sagittal scan (fat suppression technique). Reactive hyperemia of calcaneus at the Achilles tendon insertion

formed, because it represents the only technique capable of determining the insertional bone involvement appearing as medullary edema within the bone in high contrast sequences (Fig. 4.42).

A peculiar form of enthesopathy is that affecting patients in adolescence. During growth, the tendon insertion does not occur on the bone, but on the growth plate cartilage, that represents a weaker structure of the enthesis compared to bone and tendon, and is less resistant to mechanical stress. Impact is therefore mostly absorbed by the growth plate cartilage, and the corresponding bone and tendon are relatively spared. Typical clinical conditions that follow this situation are some juvenile osteochondroses, such as Osgood-Schlatter's disease (affecting the patellar tendon at its distal insertion), Sinding-Larsen-Johansson's disease (affecting the patellar tendon at its proximal insertion) and Haglund-Sever's disease (affecting the Achilles). All these patients present with pain at the enthesis level and functional loss. The typical US pattern shows thickened growth plate cartilage and fragmented nucleus of ossification, suggestive of irregular enchondral ossification [53, 54] (Fig. 4.43 a,b).

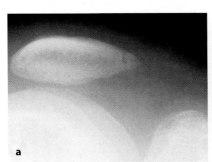

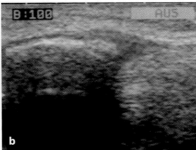

Fig. 4.43 a, b

Sinding-Larsen-Johansson syndrome in a young patient. **a** The plain film shows fragmented appearance of the ossification centre of the lower patellar pole. **b** The US scan shows an irregular bone outline and swelling at the patellar tendon insertion

Tendon tears

A tendon tear may be observed after an acute injury or as a poor outcome of tendinosis, with a spontaneous rupture. Mechanical overload, especially when excessive and repetitive, may eventually cause partial or total tears within a degenerative tendon structure. Such tears are often incomplete, but they still alter the tendon continuity and, consequently, its integrity. Histological samples show degenerative involution of the collagen fibers,

with necrotic foci. On US scans, a tear appears as a hypo to anechoic spot that interrupts the fibrillar structure of the tendon (Fig. 4.44 a, b). In complete tears, US allows the discontinuity of the fibers, the two tendon stumps and the hemorragic collection within the retraction gap to be visualized [14-16, 55]. In these cases it is important to perform a dynamic US examination for a more accurate evaluation of the tear location.

In some regions, the US signs of tendon tears can be very complicated. A clear example is represented

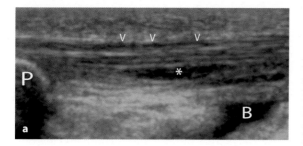

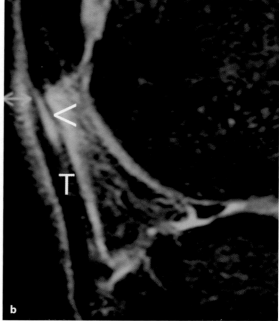

Fig. 4.44 a, b

a This longitudinal scan at the proximal third of patellar tendon shows a partial tear (*) with inflammatory involvement of peritenon (*arrowheads*). P = lower patellar extremity; B = deep pretibial bursa. **b** The MR scan of the same patient (sagittal scan, fat suppression technique) confirms the US findings and highlights the inflammation of peritendinous tissues. T = patellar tendon; *arrowheads* = partial tear

by the rotator cuff tendons and particularly by the supraspinatus tendon in which tears are classified, according to the site and extension of the lesion, into:
- *partial lesions*, these can be further divided into: *bursal*, when the involved aspect of the tendon is in contact with the subacromion-deltoid bursa (Fig. 4.45); *articular*, when the involved aspect is in contact with the humeral head and *intratendinous*. A partial intratendinous tear appears as an anechoic line within the tendon substance (Fig. 4.46).

- *complete lesions*, that correspond to full-thickness tears of the tendon (small, intermediate, wide, total) (Fig. 4.47), with possible retraction of the two stumps.

In complete lesions, the humeral head appears uncovered with a tendency to articulate with the acromion (subacromial impingement). Hypoanechoic fluid collection is observed between the two tendon stumps with a consequent expansion of the subacromion-deltoid bursa [56-59] (Fig. 4.48 a, b).

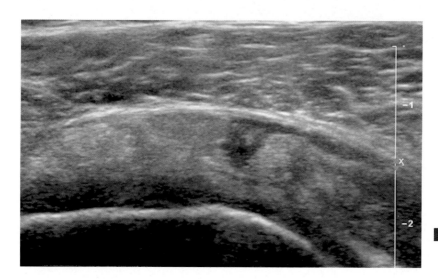

Fig. 4.45

Partial tear of bursal side of supraspinatus tendon

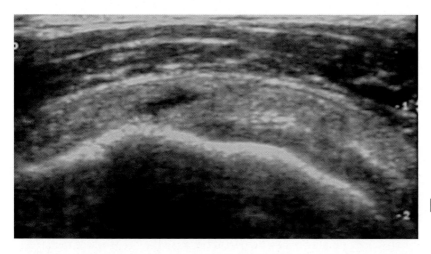

Fig. 4.46

Partial tear of supraspinatus tendon

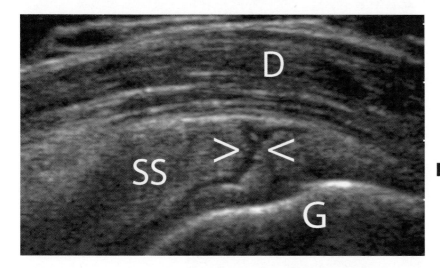

Fig. 4.47

Complete tear of supraspinatus tendon (*arrowheads*) is clearly shown as a full thickness rupture in this US scan. *SS* = supraspinatus tendon; *D* = deltoid; *G* = greater humeral tubercle

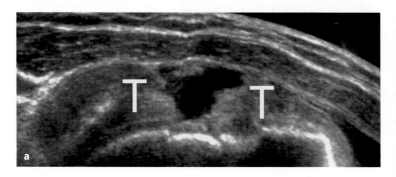

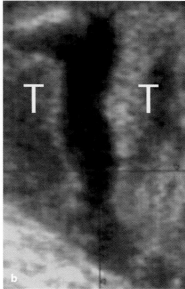

Fig. 4.48 a, b

a Complete tear of a degenerative supraspinatus tendon with retraction of the two tendon stumps. **b** MPR reconstruction on a coronal plan (*view from the top*). *T* = tendon stumps

Tendon dislocations

Along their course, sliding tendons may undergo flexion and consequent spatial misalignment from the corresponding muscle's functional axis. In order for correct biomechanical function, the angular points and lever fulcri of the tendon must be kept in their physiological osteo-fibrous grooves. The anatomic structures that carry out this task are the *retinacula* – focal transverse thickenings of the deep fascia that are securely anchored to bone eminences. The correct functioning of their stabilizing role is therefore of great importance because whenever it is lacking, the tendon tends to dislocate, with consequent instability. There are several degrees of severity in tendon instability: in moderate lesions the tendon tends to dislocate only when a specific movement is performed, while in more severe lesions subluxation and luxation can be observed. The possibility of performing dynamic examination makes US the gold standard technique when tendon instability is suspected.

Even though tendon instability is not very common, it should always be considered when deriving a differential diagnosis, because an early diagnosis is fundamental to avoid the onset of tendinosis or of a tendon tear. The most com-monly affected tendons are the long head of the brachial biceps at the shoulder and the fibular tendons at the ankle.

Dislocation of the long head of biceps may follow a transverse ligament tear or a coraco-humeral ligament tear, with or without an associated tear of the subscapularis tendon [60]. It should be mentioned that there are several congenital conditions that promote instability, such as the presence of a flat intertubercular groove. When dislocation occurs, US shows an empty groove and a medially dislocated tendon (Fig. 4.49). The application of dynamic maneuvers with external rotation of the arm, with 90° flexion of the elbow, can be useful because they reproduce the stressing action [61-64].

At the ankle, the fibular tendons are kept in site by the fibular retinacula, superior and inferior, that are respectively located over and under the angular flexion point, at the lateral malleolus [65]. Instability is caused by a lesion of the superior fibular retinaculum with subsequent tendency of the fibular tendons to dislocate anteriorly over the lateral malleolus. In short axis views, with the transducer on the angular flexion point and performing a dynamic maneuver of dorsal flexion of the foot, dislocation of the fibular tendons over the lateral malleolus can be observed (Fig. 4.50 a, b).

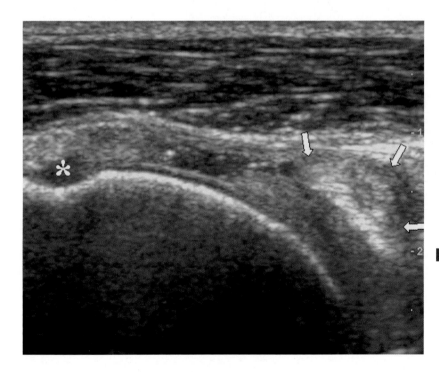

Fig. 4.49

Transverse scan of the anterior aspect of the shoulder. A complete medial dislocation of long head of biceps tendon is shown (*arrows*), caused by a complete tear of sub-scapularis tendon. The inter-tuber-cular groove is empty (*)

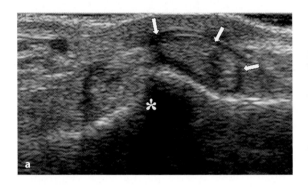

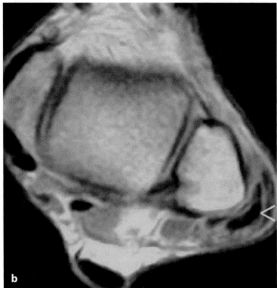

Fig. 4.50 a, b

a Lateral compartment of ankle, transverse scan. Dislocation of fibular tendons (*arrows*) over the fibular malleolus (*) is shown. **b** MR scan in the same patient (axial scan, SE T1W sequence) confirm the fibular tendons luxation (*arrowhead*)

Tendon cysts

Tendon cysts occur more frequently in the palmar aspect of fingers, along the flexor tendons course, strictly in contact with the tenosynovial sheath from which they arise. The US diagnosis is simple because they usually appear as round, anechoic, formations with well-defined walls [1, 14, 15, 44]. They should always be evaluated in long and short axis views (Fig.4.51 a, b); short axis views allow the relation between cyst and tenosynovial sheath to be demonstrated. A dynamic examination can be performed during flexion of the fingers.

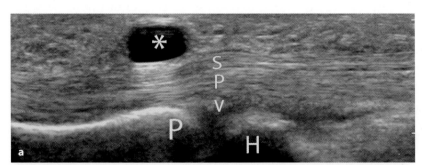

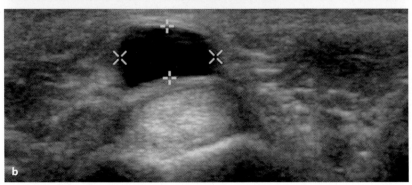

Fig. 4.51 a, b

a Longitudinal scan of a finger. An anechoic tendon cyst (*) is shown. Note the typical anechoic appearance and the dorsal acoustic enhancement. *s* = flexor superficialis tendon; *p* = flexor profundus tendon; *v* = volar plate; *P* = base of proximal phalanx; *H* = metacarpal head. **b** Transverse scan of the same patient that allows the relationship between the cyst (calipers) and the tendon sheath to be visualized

Ligament tears

Compared to tendons, ligaments are thinner and contain a higher amount of elastin, to give a better stabilization of the joints with the necessary elasticity. There are two different types of ligaments: *intrinsic capsular ligaments*, consisting of focal thickenings of the articular capsule with a strengthening function, and *extrinsic ligaments*, which do not depend on the capsule and can be further divided into *extracapsular* and *intracapsular*.

US can easily assess the ligaments of the medial and lateral compartment of the ankle (deltoid, anterior talofibular and calcaneofibular), the collateral ligaments of the knee, the collateral and annular ligaments of the elbow, the coraco-acromial and coraco-humeral ligaments of the shoulder, and the ulnar collateral ligament of the first metacarpo-phalangeal joint [66].

When assessing a ligament tear, it should always be remembered that US, unlike MR, is limited by its small field of view that does not allow an overview of the joint compartments. US, therefore, is not able to detect a possible concomitant lesion of the joint, which is a fundamental diagnosis in order to plan correct therapy.

Ligaments are mainly affected by traumatic injuries that can be classified as 1st degree (stretching lesions), 2nd degree (partial lesions) and 3rd degree (complete lesions). They can be divided into acute, subacute and chronic. It should be kept in mind that the US assessment of a ligament injury can be more accurate when performed a few days after the trauma, in a subacute phase. Only then does the enzymatic lysis of figurative elements cause a progressive reduction of the echoes and of the corpuscular appearance of the haemorrhagic effusion. Finally, the collection appears anechoic and it is used as acoustic window to visualize the ligament lesion.

In *1st degree injuries*, US shows a thickened ligament with a relatively hypoechoic appearance, depending on the interstitial edema; the ligament is continuous with a regular outline (Fig. 4.52 a, b).

In *2nd degree injuries* the normal echotexture appears altered. The ligament is thickened, inhomogeneous and shows an irregular outline; a minimal discontinuity of the ligament can be observed.

In *3rd degree injuries*, US allows a full thickness lesion to be detected, with possible retraction of the fibers and the haemorrhagic collection filling the gap (Fig. 4.53 a, b). A dynamic examination is always useful in doubtful cases.

To assess subacute and acute ligament injuries,

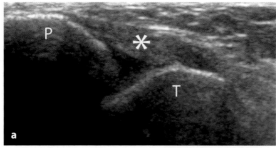

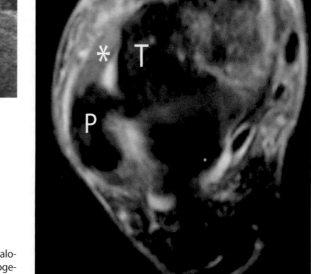

Fig. 4.52 a, b

a US scan of lateral compartment of ankle. The anterior talofibular ligament is continuous but thickened and inhomogeneous for a 1st degree lesion. **b** MR axial scan in the same patient (fat suppression technique). *P* = fibula; *T* = talus

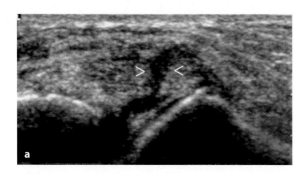

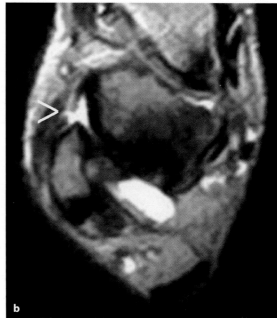

Fig. 4.53 a, b

a US scan of lateral compartment of ankle. The anterior talo-fibular ligament is completely torn (*arrowheads*) with abundant effusion. **b** MR scan in the same patient (axial scan, TSE T2W). *Arrowhead* = tear

power Doppler analysis allows the presence of diffuse perilesional hyperemia to be detected.

In the presence of fibrous and scar tissue resulting from a post-traumatic ligament lesion, US shows typically focal hypoechoic tissue. In some cases, minute calcification can also be found.

4.4 Muscles

In spite of US being considered the gold standard for the diagnosis of muscle pathology, it has a very important role and should be considered the first choice imaging technique. When an inflammatory, degenerative or a malignant pathology is in progress, US must be complemented with computed tomography (CT) or MR, while in the cases of trauma it is mostly exhaustive.

According to etiology, muscular pathology can be divided into:
- inflammatory and degenerative;
- malignant;
- traumatic (major and minor lesions).

Rheumatology mostly deals with inflammatory and degenerative pathology, but a deep knowledge of the other lesions is necessary for a correct differential diagnosis.

Degenerative muscular pathology does not show any specific features within the echotextures, but it is possible to detect some characteristic ultrasound signs of degeneration in several inflammatory pathologies. Myositis shows a diffuse reduction in the echogenicity of the tissues that is directly proportional to the amount of inflammatory edema in the fibrillar muscular structure.

Muscular inflammatory pathology

Muscular inflammatory pathology can be divided into:
- non-specific myositis (serous, purulent and chronic);
- specific myositis (syphilitic, tubercular and viral);
- focal myositis ossificans (post-traumatic, post-inflammatory and chronic);
- interstitial granulomatous myositis of unknown origin;
- polymyositis.

Serous myositis has a traumatic, toxi-infective or viral origin. It is characterized by interstitial inflammatory, hyperemia and serous infiltration of the perimysium. The thickening of the muscle fascicles is a typical degenerative after-effect. In the earlier stages, the muscular structure can be easily assessed with US and it appears thickened and diffusely hypoechoic, due to the perimysial edema, with hazy muscular fascicles that appear interrupted and spaced (Fig. 4.54). In the later stages, fibro-adipose involution has an inhomogeneous appearance.

Purulent myositis, usually caused by deep and infected wounds or by blood flow-derived bacteria, is characterized by several scattered abscessed foci. With US, the abscess appears as a hypo-anechoic rounded mass, with hazy margins and inhomogeneous echoes [67]. This kind of examination allows the size and the site of the abscess to be precisely described and a percutaneous drainage of the purulent material to be performed. In the later stages, the echogenicity of the abscess either further reduces or, if they become chronic, increases according to the inner organization of the collection (filaments, fibrous branches or sediments) with a consensual hyperechoic appearance of the wall (pseudocapsular appearance) [68].

Chronic myositis, follows an acute non-specific myositis, is characterized by fibrosclerotic substitution of the normal echotexture with an increase of the interstitial connective tissue that can also involve large parts of the muscle belly.

Tubercular myositis is usually the result of direct propagation of bone, articular or lymphoglandular granulomas; the caseous exudate spreads through the interstitium to the muscular tissue, producing complex and extensive fistulous tracts. Haematogeneous tubercular dissemination in patients affected by miliary tuberculosis is extremely rare.

The most common *viral myositis* is caused by Coxsackie B virus (Bornholm's disease), and is characterized by necrotic and degenerative lesions of the muscle fibers.

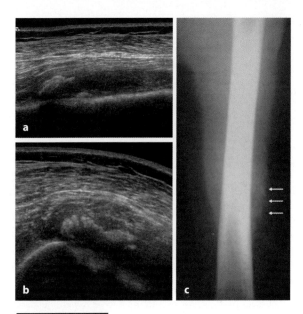

Fig. 4.55 a-c

Ultrasound of thigh on longitudinal (**a**) and axial (**b**) views showing the evolution towards a myositis ossificans, with blurred calcified spots in the muscle. **c** Corresponding plain radiograph showing mild blurry calcifications (*arrows*) within soft tissues close to femoral diaphysis

Myositis ossificans may have different forms: *focal myositis ossificans* can represent the fibro-calcific involution following violent trauma, chronic inflammatory processes or suppurative lesions, or it can be the direct consequence of central or peripheral nervous system diseases. Sometimes, it can represent natural evolution of an intramuscular hematoma that calcifies and leads to an ossification process (Fig. 4.55 a-c); the development of these lesions occurs over a five-six months period.

In earlier phases, the lesion has an inhomogeneous architecture and may mimic neoplasia; afterwards, the first calcification appears, mostly on the margins, which is then followed by true ossification (Fig. 4.56).

Progressive Myositis Ossificans (PMO) or Progressive Ossificans Fibrodysplasia of Munchmeyer is a rare and incurable genetic disease with autosomal dominant transmission, characterized by a progressive ossification of skeletal muscles until a complete substitution with a mineralized osseous matrix has occured. The early histopathologic alterations of connective tissue (particularly aponeurosis, fascias, tendons and ligaments) represent the

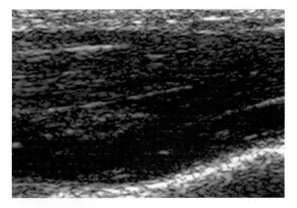

Fig. 4.54

Serous myositis. The muscle appear thickened and hypoechoic in relation to an extensive perimysial edema

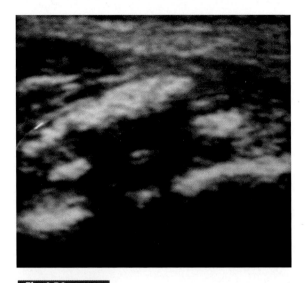

Fig. 4.56

Advanced myositis ossificans, with multiple foci of calcification within the muscle

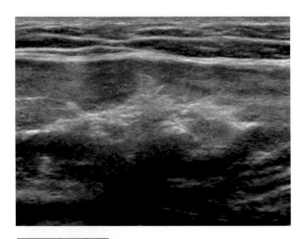

Fig. 4.57

Extensive muscular fibrosis with multiple fibrocalcific areas within the muscle

basics of the disease, while skeletal muscle is involved last. At first, US shows typical muscular inflammation, with reduced echoes within the involved areas; then the consequent fibrous involution causes a hypoechoic appearance (Fig. 4.57) until several ossified foci can be observed in later stages. In these cases, other imaging techniques are necessary to understand the exact origin of the bony growths [69].

Polymyositis consists of a group of muscular disorders of unknown origin characterized by an inflammatory process of the skeletal musculature. Polymyositis is classified among the systemic rheumatic diseases, more precisely among the connective tissue diseases, and can be idiopathic, juvenile or tumor-related. The main symptom is muscular weakness that mainly affects the proximal muscles of the limb girdle musculature. Several cutaneous symptoms are characteristically associated with this disease. US is helpful both as a diagnostic tool, detecting the muscular degeneration areas and the intramuscular calcific foci, and as a guide to muscular biopsy, which is necessary to definitively confirm the diagnosis [70].

Muscular neoplastic pathology

Space-occupying lesions of muscle may arise from the striated muscular fibrocells or from the components of the connective tissue.

Benign tumors may be located in one or more muscle bellies and usually have sharp borders, regular margins and homogeneous echotexture. Usually, they do not have an infiltrative appearance but they rather seem to be expansile masses that spread and displace the muscular fibers and the connective branches, leaving them intact. Therefore, the epimysium is spared and remains continuous in every part and, upon dynamic assessment, the muscular bellies slide regularly onto the adjacent structures (Fig. 4.58 a-c).

Nevertheless, there are some muscular lesions, mostly smaller than 3 or 4 cm, which show benign echotexture, but then turn out to be malignant after histological examination. Even though US can provide relevant information about the nature of the neoplasm (fibromas appear hyperechoic compared to the muscle, while lipomas may appear weakly hyperechoic or even hypoechoic), the role of color Doppler is very important, as well as the use of US contrast media that can provide further elements for the benign or malignant characterization of lesions. For instance, a vascular pattern with regular architecture, with one or two vascular pedicles and with characteristic wash-in and wash-out curves (Fig. 4.59 a-c) can lead to the diagnosis of a benign neoplasm [71, 72].

Malignant tumors, when they are not small, have an irregular shape with hazy and ill-defined borders (Fig. 4.60), with inhomogeneous echo-

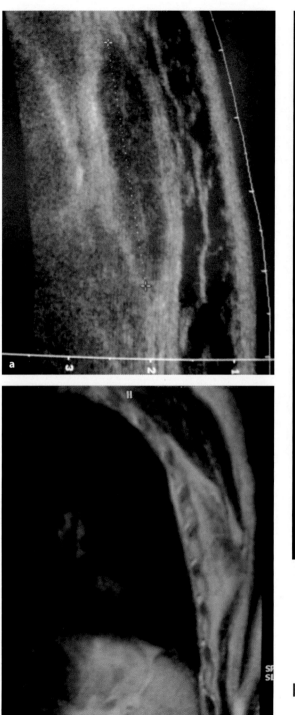

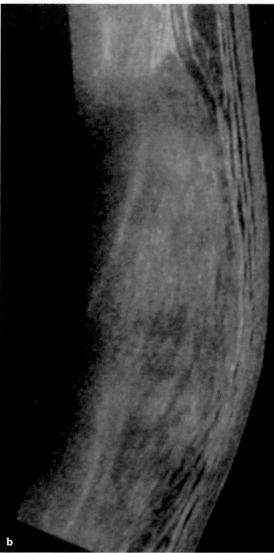

Fig. 4.58 a–c

Elastofibroma of the back. It appears homogeneously hypoe-choic (**a**) or inhomogeneously hyperechoic (**b**). **c** MR scan (SE T1W sequence) corresponding to the US image (**b**)

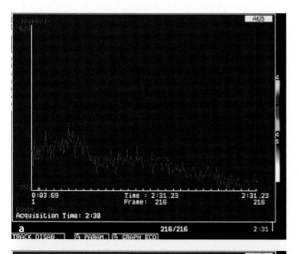

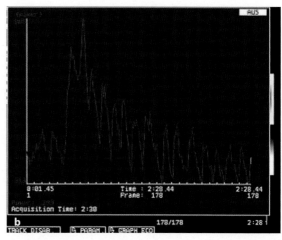

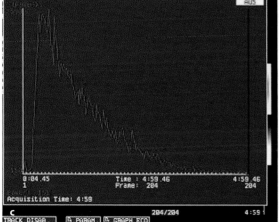

Fig. 4.59 a-c

Wash-in and wash-out graphs of vascular enhancement after contrast agent: (**a**) lipoma; (**b**) leiomyosarcoma; (**c**) synovial sarcoma (courtesy of Carlo Faletti, MD)

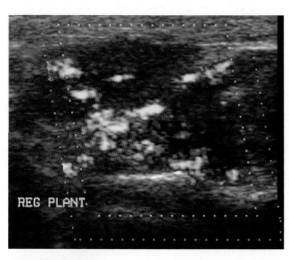

Fig. 4.60

The power Doppler scan shows a hypoechoic mass, with irregular contour and disorganised vascular pattern

texture due to the presence of anechoic areas caused by necrosis. The epimysium is frequently interrupted and invaded: for this reason, the dynamic assessment shows an alteration of the sliding of muscular bellies on the surrounding structures.

Blood borne metastases are uncommon but maintain the malignant characteristics of the primitive lesion. Nevertheless, if the metastasis is small, it can assume some benign features. Moreover, a metastatic deposition contiguous with the muscular fascia and the epimysium can occur, for instance, in the pectoralis major muscle when it is infiltrated by breast cancer at a late stage. In these cases, the muscle does not have any cleavage from the original neoplasm and appears retracted on superficial and deep planes. Another cause of muscle tumour is a hyatid cyst which is very uncommon and the ultrasound appearance is the same as in the liver. US is very effective at differentiating cysts, often multiloculated with several septa, from other expansile lesions [73] (Fig. 4.61). In these cases, US is extremely helpful in performing US-guided interventions.

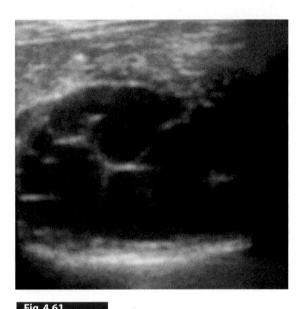

Fig. 4.61

US scan of multiloculated hydatid cysts presenting internal thick septa

Muscular traumatic pathology

US is extremely helpful in the field of muscular trauma.

Within *minor traumatic lesions*, muscular contractures and contusions are difficult to detect with US, unless complemented with an accurate comparative examination. They are characterized by slight widening of perimysial partitions with hypoechoic post-traumatic edema. *Major traumatic lesions* are represented by intramuscular *hematoma* and *muscle rupture*.

Muscular hematoma is the typical sign of a muscular tear and its dimensions usually indicate the extension of the tear (excluding some hematological conditions). The formation of a hematoma creates dissection of the fascial planes and, if the collection exceeds 100 ml of fluid – as in case of a complete rupture – it must be drained quickly to avoid any compression on the surrounding muscular and neurovascular structures (Fig. 4.62).

The evolution of an intramuscular hematoma is not dissimilar to that which occurs in other sites of the human body. A recent hemorrhage has a hyperechoic appearance (Fig. 4.63) but becomes hypoechoic after a couple of hours until a separation between the liquid and the corpuscular phase occurs. When the hematoma is resolving, it appears as a homogeneous anechoic collection (Fig. 4.64 a, b) that can be more or less organized [14, 15, 74].

Muscular ruptures can be caused by compression (direct trauma) or by a distraction of the mus-

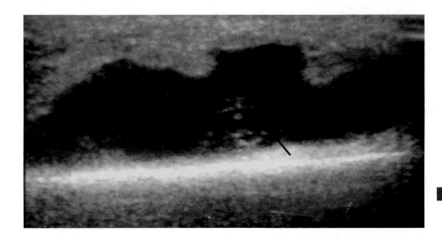

Fig. 4.62

Extensive muscle effusion comprised of serous fluid and blood

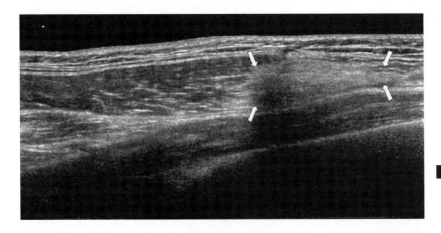

Fig. 4.63

Diffusely hyperechoic hematoma (*arrows*) following recent muscle trauma

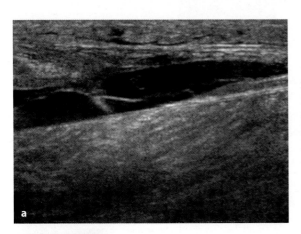

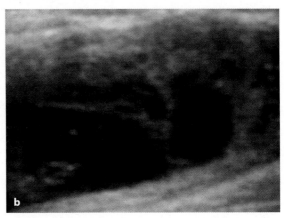

Fig. 4.64 a, b

a Deep hematoma at early stage with internal thin septa. **b** Hematoma at a later stage: the septa appear thicker

cular extremities. If direct trauma occurs, the muscle is directly compressed against the underlying bone. US demonstrates an irregular cavity with rough borders followed, a few hours after the trauma, by a hematoma. As the lesion heals, US can detect extensive cicatricial tissue that appears hyperechoic and calcific (post-traumatic myositis ossificans).

Indirect trauma is caused by a sudden and violent contraction of the muscle and is more frequent in the lower limbs, especially in those muscles that connect two bone segments.

Distraction traumas can be divided into three groups, according to their ultrasound features: strain (grade I), partial rupture (grade II) and complete rupture (grade III).

Muscle strain occurs when it is stretched beyond its elastic limit. The patient reports acute pain that cannot be distinguished from cramp. The lesions are mostly microscopic but the macroscopic exam can detect several small sero-hemorragic collections up to 6-7 centimeters long and from 2-10 millimeters of diameter. On US, these collections have a stretched and irregular hypoechoic appearance. Healing occurs in about two weeks.

Partial rupture (grade II) is a lesion that occurs when the muscle is stretched over its maximal elastic potential. It involves more than 5% of the muscular tissue but not the whole transverse section. In acute cases, the patient reports a 'snap' with localised sharp pain and a complete loss of muscle function that is usually recovered in a couple of days. US clearly shows the discontinuity of the muscle with interruption of the fibroadipose septa, in particular at the myotendinous junction, as in the gastrocnemius [14, 15, 74] (Fig. 4.65 a, b).

A partial rupture shows three different US findings: a hypoechoic cavity within the muscular tissue, a thick hyperechoic cavity border and the 'bell-clapper' sign, due to small shreds of muscular tissue floating in the hematoma [14, 15, 74] (Fig. 4.66).

Complete ruptures (grade III) are far less common than the other lesions. The initial clinical presentation is very similar to the partial rupture but the functional loss persists longer and, if the muscle is superficial, the lesion can be appreciated on palpation. US shows complete dislocation of the muscular ends with a hematoma filling the gap (Fig. 4.67).

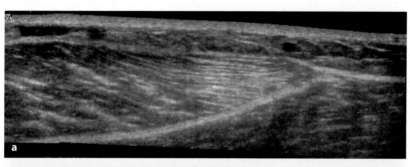

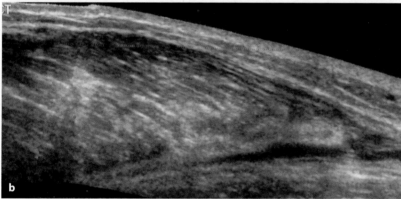

Fig. 4.65 a, b

a Normal appearance of myotendinous junction of medial gastrocnemius. **b** Partial tear of medial gastrocnemius at the myotendinous junction

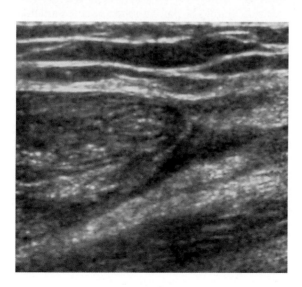

Fig. 4.66

Bell-clapper appearance of muscular stump

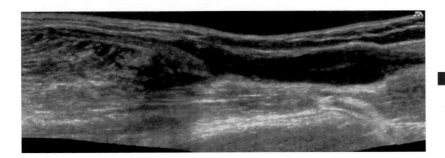

Fig. 4.67

Complete rupture of rectus femoris with dimpling of muscular stumps and wide sero-hemorragic collection filling the resulting gap

Role of Doppler techniques

In healthy subjects, Doppler techniques are able to assess the vascularization of muscles, detecting both arteries and veins (Fig. 4.68). This is direct-

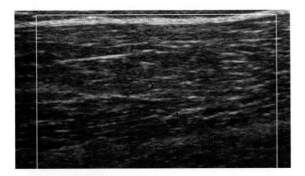

Fig. 4.68

US of resting muscle, normal appearance

ly related to the sensitivity of the equipment. Depending on the type and generation of the US equipment, several differences can be observed in the evaluation of the vascularization of the same anatomical region. Some recent studies have demonstrated how, during physical strain, color Doppler is able to demonstrate an increase in the muscle vascularization thanks to local hyperemia and to the opening of several arteriovenous shunts, whose purpose is to increase the metabolic exchanges of the involved muscular cells [75] (Fig. 4.69 a, b).

Doppler is not used as a routine analysis during US examination of muscle but it can be used to assess the vascularization of neoplasms. Some recent studies have identified the existence of several vascular patterns which increase diagnostic reliability for the characterization of expansive lesions [75, 76].

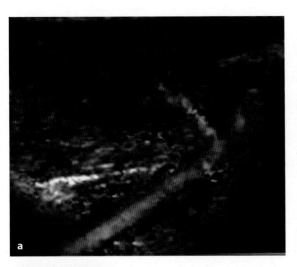
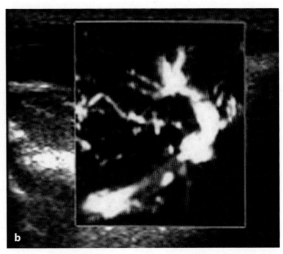

Fig. 4.69 a, b

a Color-Doppler scan of muscle after exercise, normal appearance. **b** In the same muscle, power Doppler allows a more detailed assessment of vascular network

4.5 Nerves

In entrapment neuropathies, extrinsic pressure causes demyelination, axonal degeneration, intranervous venous congestion and edema. These changes may either regress after removal of the compressive agent or progress toward intraneural fibrosis, leading to permanent loss of nerve function and atrophy of the innervated muscles. US signs include changes in both nerve shape and echotexture, the most common being a sudden flattening (notch sign) with focal reduction in the nerve cross-sectional area at the compression point and the nerve swelling that occurs proximal to the level of compression. The nerve swelling is typically fusiform, extending 2-4 cm in length, and appears maximal in close proximity to the compression level. Based on these features, US has proven to be an accurate means for identifying the level of compression. Although nerve flattening should be regarded as the main sign of nerve compression, quantitative analysis of nerve thickening by means of the ellipse formula [(maximum AP diameter) x (maximum LL diameter) x ($\pi/4$)] has proved to be the most consistent criterion for the diagnosis at various entrapment sites [77]. With respect to electrophysiological findings, a positive correlation was found between the nerve cross-sectional area and the severity of electromyographic findings, whereas only a modest negative correlation seems to exist between elec-

trodiagnostic parameters, such as motor velocity, compound motor action potential (CMAP) amplitude, distal sensory nerve action potential (SNAP), and the nerve cross-sectional area [78, 79]. It is conceivable that loss of axons may be associated with nerve enlargement as an expression of increased amount of endoneurial edema.

In entrapment neuropathies, the nerve echotexture may become uniformly hypoechoic with loss of the fascicular pattern at the level of the compression site and proximal to it. In general, the hypoechoic changes in the epineurium of compressed nerves occur gradually and become more severe as the nerve progresses toward the site of compression. Depiction of such changes may increase the confidence in the diagnosis and in determining the level of the entrapment. An enhanced depiction of intraneural blood flow signals can also be appreciated with color and power Doppler techniques as a sign of local disturbances in the nerve microvasculature that occur in a compressive context.

Another common pathological condition which represents a peculiar kind of nerve compression seems to be the case of the Morton neuroma (Fig. 4.70 a-c).

This forefoot lesion is related to chronic compression and repeated microtrauma on the interdigital nerves at the level of the distal edge of the intermetatarsal ligament. These lesions most frequently occur within the second or third interspace

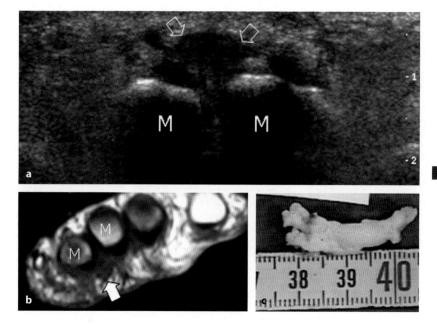

Fig. 4.70 a-c

Morton neuroma. **a** Transverse 12-5MHz US image obtained over the plantar aspect of the metatarsal heads with T1-weighted MR imaging correlation (**b**) demonstrates a solid hypoechoic mass (*arrows*) consistent with a Morton neuroma between the third and fourth metatarsals (M). **c** Surgical specimen

and lead to development of a fusiform hypoechoic mass elongated along the major axis of the metatarsals [80-82]. US has a reported 95-100% sensitivity, 83% specificity and 95% accuracy in the diagnosis of Morton neuromas [83]. Longitudinal scans may demonstrate the continuity of the mass with the interdigital nerve. Missing neuromas are related to suboptimal experience of the examiner and to the small size of the lesion. The coexistence of an enlarged intermetatarsal bursa can explain the mixed or anechoic appearance of some lesions and their extension dorsal to the plantar aspect of metatarsals [83].

4.6 Dermis and hypodermis

Assessment of skin and subcutaneous tissue is possible using high frequency transducers (up to 30 MHz), that are able to differentiate skin from subcutaneous tissue. Specific skin disease is usually diagnosed by clinical examination sometimes followed by skin biopsy.

Currently US has no role in the diagnosis of skin lesions but can be very helpful in assessing and following up several systemic pathologies with cutaneous involvement.

In *dermatopolymyositis*, cutaneous lesions can be easily found; for example the characteristic Gottron's papule, erythematous or violaceous plaques,

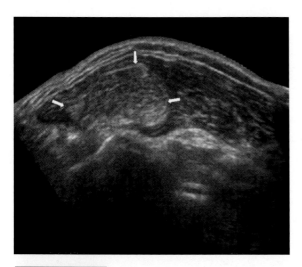

Fig. 4.71

Transverse US scan depicting an inhomogeneously hyperechoic nodular mass (*arrows*) related to a superficial lipoma, which is located within subcutaneous tissue of elbow

slightly thickened over bony eminences, often detected on the extensor aspect of fingers joints. With US they appear as small nodular iso-hyperechoic areas with characteristic calcification if the disease occurs in childhood. Involvement of adipose tissue is observed as moderate thickening that appears as a homogeneous hyperechoic line affecting of the fibrous connective tissue bands that lose their linear architecture [84].

On US, *liposclerosis* is characterized by hypoechoic micro- and macronodules of fibrous tissue that progressively replace the subcutaneous tissue.

Rheumatic nodules have a hypoechoic appearance with smooth margins and can be sometimes mistaken for gout tophi; the incidental finding of calcific intralesional foci (hyperechoic with posterior acoustic shadow) makes the diagnosis easier [85].

In *systemic sclerosis*, sclero-atrophic hypo-isoechoic alteration of the subcutaneous tissue can be seen, especially in the finger-tips.

Subcutaneous edema is characterized by a large-mesh hypoechoic net with a characteristic 'cobblestone' appearance.

Panniculitis is an inflammatory phenomenon of the subcutaneous tissue with a probable vasculitic origin. It can be divided into lobular and septal panniculitis and appear as hypo-hyperechoic inhomogeneous areas, rich in calcific nodules of various dimensions (1 cm up to 15 cm in erythema nodosum). Moreover, in the acute phases, marked surrounding edema and thickening of the septa can be seen.

Lipomas and *angiomas* are common findings and are characterized by specific US vascular pattern [14, 15, 86] (Figs. 4.71, 4.72 a, b).

There are several pathologies – less important but not less common – involving the overloaded fat pads in specific anatomical sites, such as the fibro-adipose subcalcanear sole, that may be affected in overload syndromes that involve the nearby plantar fascia (Fig. 4.73).

Plantar fibromatosis (*Ledderhose disease*) is a pathological condition characterized by nodularity along the aponeurosis course which appears homogeneously hypoechoic (Fig. 4.74 a, b) and shows no vascular signals at color and power Doppler analysis [87].

A similar condition, sometimes connected with plantar fibromatosis, is *Dupuytren's contracture*, in which the hypoechoic nodules are found in longitudinal bundles of the palmar fascia along the course of the flexor tendons [88].

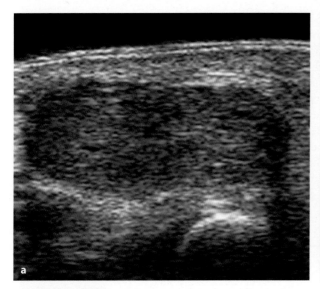
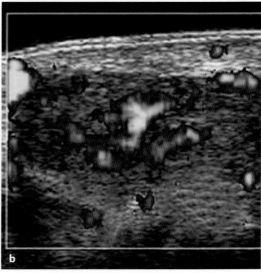

Fig. 4.72 a, b

a Hypoechoic, ovoid, well-defined mass typical of an angioma. **b** The corresponding power Doppler scan shows the typical vascular pattern with a single pedicle

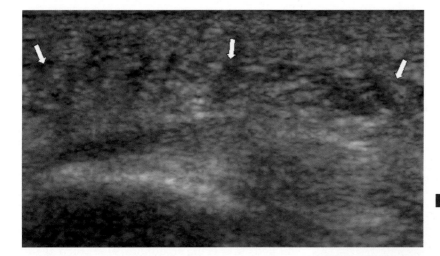

Fig. 4.73

Plantar fascitis. Inhomogeneous appearance of subcutaneous planes (*arrows*)

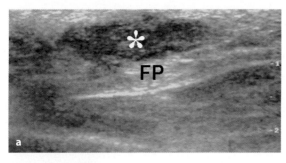
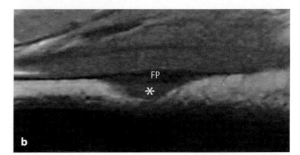

Fig. 4.74 a, b

a Plantar side of foot, longitudinal US scan. A hypoechoic subcutaneous nodule (*) is found adjacent to the plantar fascia. **b** MR sagittal scan of the same patient confirming the finding (*). *FP* = plantar fascia

References

1. Grassi W, Cervini C (1998) Ultrasonography in rheumatology: an evolving technique. Ann Rheum Dis 57:268-271
2. Grassi W, Filippucci E, Farina A (2005) Ultrasonography in osteoarthritis. Semin Arthritis Rheum 34:19-23
3. Grassi W, Tittarelli E, Pirani O et al (1993) Ultrasound examination of metacarpophalangeal joints in rheumatoid arthritis. Scand J Rheumatol 22:243-247
4. Grassi W, Lamanna G, Farina A, Cervini C (1999) Sonographic imaging of normal and osteoarthritic cartilage. Semin Arthritis Rheum 28:398-403
5. Grassi W, Salaffi F, Filippucci E (2005) Ultrasound in rheumatology. Best Pract Res Clin Rheumatol 19:467-485
6. Aisen AM, McCune WJ, MacGuire A et al (1984) Sonographic evaluation of the cartilage of the knee. Radiology 102:781-784
7. McCune WJ, Dedrock DK, Aisen AM, MacGuire A (1990) Sonographic evaluation of osteoarthritic femoral condylar cartilage. Correlation with operative findings. Clin Orthop 254:230-235
8. Grassi W, Tittarelli E, Cervini C (1993) L'ecotomografia nella gonartrosi. Il Reumatologo 14:22-26
9. Richardson ML, Selby B, Montana MA, Mack LA (1988) Ultrasonography of the knee. Radiol Clin North Am 26:63-75
10. Iagnocco A, Coari G, Zoppini A (1992) Sonographic evaluation of femoral condylar cartilage in osteoarthritis and rheumatoid arthritis. Scand J Rheumatol 21:201-203
11. Grassi W, Filippucci E, Busilacchi P (2004) Musculoskeletal ultrasound. Best Pract Res Clin Rheumatol 18:813-826
12. Martino F, Monetti G (1993) Semeiotica ecografica delle malattie reumatiche. Piccin ed., Padova
13. Frediani B, Filippou G, Falsetti P et al (2005) Diagnosis of calcium pyrophosphate dihydrate crystal deposition disease: ultrasonographic criteria proposed. Ann Rheum Dis 64:638-640
14. Van Holsbeeck MT, Introcaso JH (2001) Musculoskeletal ultrasound, 2nd edition, Mosby
15. Gibbon WW, Wakefield RJ (1999) Ultrasound in inflammatory disease. Radiol Clin North Am 37:633-651
16. Gibbon WW (2004) Applications of ultrasound in arthritis. Semin Musculoskelet Radiol 8:313-328
17. Newman JS, Adler R, Bude RO, Rubin J (1994) Detection of soft-tissue hyperemia: value of power Doppler sonography. AJR 163:385-389
18. Silvestri E, Martinoli C, Onetto F et al (1994) Valutazione dell'artrite reumatoide del ginocchio con color Doppler. Radiol Med 88:364-367
19. Carotti M, Salaffi F, Manganelli P et al (2002) Power Doppler sonography in the assessment of synovial tissue of the knee joint in reumathoid arthritis: a preliminary experience. Ann Rheum Dis 61:877-882
20. Schmidt WA, Volker L, Zacher J et al (2000) Colour Doppler ultrasonography to detect pannus in kneejoint synovitis. Clin Exp Rheumatol 18:439-444
21. Fitzgerald O, Bresnihan B (1992) Synovial vascularity is increased in rheumatoid arthritis: comment on the article by Stivens et al (letter). Arthritis Rheum 35:1540-1541
22. Walsh DA (1999) Angiogenesis and arthritis. Rheumatology 38:103-112
23. Klauser A, Frauscher F, Schirmer M et al (2002) The value of contrast enhanced color Doppler ultrasound in the detection of vascularization of finger joint in patients with rheumatoid arthritis. Arthritis Rheum 46:647-653
24. Szkudlarek M, Court-Payen M, Strandberg C et al (2000) contrast enhanced power Doppler ultrasound examination of metacarpophalangeal joints in patients with Rheumatoid Arthritis. Ann Rheum Dis 59 (Suppl 1)
25. Klauser A, Demharten J, De Marchi A et al (2005) Contrast enhanced gray-scale sonography in assessment of joint vascularity in rheumatoid arthritis: result from the IACUS study group. Eur Radiol 15:2404-2410
26. Martino F, Angelelli G, Ettorre GC et al (1992) Aspetto normale della borsa sovrarotulea nell'ecografia del ginocchio. Radiol Med 83:43-48
27. Van Holsbeeck M, Strouse PJ (1993) Sonography of the shoulder: evaluation of the subacromial-subdeltoid bursa. AJR 160:561-564
28. Fornage BD, Schernberg FL, Rifkin MD (1985) Ultrasound examination of the hand. Radiology 155:785-788
29. Steiner E, Steinbach LS, Schnarkowski P et al (1996) Ganglia and cysts around joints. Radiol Clin North Am 34:395-425
30. De Flaviis L, Musso MG (1995) Hand and wrist. Clin Diagn Ultrasound 30:151-178
31. Cardinal E, Buckwalter KA, Braunstein EM, Mih AD (1994) Occult dorsal carpal ganglion: comparison of US and MR imaging. Radiology 193:259-262
32. Teefey SA, Middleton WD, Patel V et al (2004) The accuracy of high-resolution ultrasound for evaluating focal lesions of the hand and wrist. J Hand Surg 29:393-399
33. Bianchi S, Martinoli C (1999) Detection of loose bodies in joints. Radiol Clin North Am 37:679-690
34. Roberts D, Miller TT, Erlanger SM (2004) Sonographic appearance of primary synovial chondromatosis of the knee. J Ultrasound Med 23:707-709
35. Puddu G, Ippolito E, Postacchini F (1976) A classification of Achilles tendon disease. Am J Sports Med 4:145-150
36. Garlaschi G, Silvestri E, Satragno L, Cimmino MA (2002) The rheumatoid hand: diagnostic imaging. Springer, Milano
37. Bianchi S, Martinoli C, Abdelwhab IF (2005) Ultrasound of tendon tears. Part 1: general considerations and upper extremity. Skeletal Radiol 34:500-512
38. Bianchi S, Poletti, PA, Martinoli C (2006) Ultrasound appearance of tendon tears. Part 2: lower extremity and myotendinous tears. Skeletal Radiol 35:63-77
39. Fredberg U, Bolvig L (2002) Significance of ultrasonographically detected asymptomatic tendinosis in the patellar and achilles tendons. Am J Sports Med 30:488-491
40. Maganaris CN, Narici MV, Almekinders LC (2004) Biomechanics and pathophysiology of overuse tendon injuries: ideas on insertional tendinopathy. Sports Med 34:1005-1017
41. Clement JP 4th, Kassarjian A, Palmer WE (2005) Synovial inflammatory processes in the hand. Eur J Radiol 56:307-318
42. Simmen BR, Gschwend N (1995) Tendon diseases in chronic rheumatoid arthritis Orthopade 24:224-236

43. Small LN, Ross JJ (2005) Suppurative tenosynovitis and septic bursitis. Infect Dis Clin North Am 19:991-1005

44. Grassi W, Tittarelli E, Pirani O et al (1995) Finger tendon involvement in rheumatoid arthritis: evaluation with high-frequency sonography. Arthritis Rheum 38:186-194

45. Nagaoka M, Matsuzaki H, Suzuki T (2000) Ultrasonographic examination of de Quervain's disease. J Orthop Sci 5:96-99

46. Giovagnorio F, Andreoli C, De Cicco ML. Ultrasonographic evaluation of de Quervain disease. J Ultrasound Med, Vol 16, Issue 10:685-689

47. Silvestri E, Biggi E, Molfetta L et al (2003) Power Doppler analysis of tendon vascularization. Int J Tissue React 25:149-158

48. Richards PJ, Win T, Jones PW (2005) The distribution of microvascular response in Achilles tendonopathy assessed by colour and power Doppler. Skeletal Radiol 34:336-342

49. Martinoli C, Derchi LE, Pastorino C et al (1993) Analysis of echotexture of tendons with US. Radiology 186:839-843

50. Ulreich N, Kainberger F, Huber W, Nehrer S (2002) Achilles tendon and sports. Radiologe 42:811-817

51. Lohrer H, Arentz S (2003) Impingement lesion of the distal anterior Achilles tendon in sub-Achilles bursitis and Haglund-pseudoexostosis-a therapeutic challenge Sportverletz Sportschaden 17:181-188

52. Terslev L, Qvistgaard E, Torp-Pedersen S et al (2001) Ultrasound and Power Doppler findings in jumper's knee - preliminary observations. Eur J Ultrasound 13:183-189

53. De Flaviis L, Nessi R, Scaglione P et al (1989) Ultrasonic diagnosis of Osgood-Schlatter and Sinding-Larsen-Johansson diseases of the knee. Skeletal Radiol 18:193-197

54. Mahlfeld K, Kayser R, Franke J, Merk H (2001) Ultrasonography of the Osgood-Schlatter disease. Ultraschall Med 22:182-185

55. Bianchi S, Cohen M, Jacob D (2005) Tendons traumatic lesions. J Radiol 86(12 Pt 2):1845-1857

56. Bouffard JA, Lee SM, Dhanju J (2000) Ultrasonography of the shoulder. Semin Ultrasound CT MR 21:164-191

57. Middleton WD, Teefey SA, Yamaguchi K (2004) Sonography of the rotator cuff: analysis of interobserver variability. AJR 183:1465-1468

58. Teefey SA, Middleton WD, Yamaguchi K (1999) Shoulder sonography: state of the art. Radiol Clin North Am 37:767-785

59. Ptasznik R (1997) Sonography of the shoulder. In: van Holsbeeck MT, Introcaso JH (eds) Musculoskeletal ultrasound. Saunders, St. Louis, pp 463-516

60. Werner A, Mueller T, Boehm D, Gohlke F (2000) The stabilizing sling for the long head of the biceps tendon in the rotator cuff interval: a histoanatomic study. Am J Sports Med 28:28-31

61. Farin PU, Jaroma H, Harju A, Soimakallio S (1995) Medial displacement of the biceps brachii tendon: evaluation with dynamic sonography during maximal external shoulder rotation. Radiology 195:845-848

62. Patton WC, McCluskey GM (2001) Biceps tendinitis and subluxation. Clin Sports Med 20:505-529

63. Ptasznik R, Hennesy O (1995) Abnormalities of the biceps tendon of the shoulder: sonographic findings. AJR 164:409-414

64. Prato N, Derchi LE, Martinoli C (1996) Sonographic diagnosis of biceps tendon dislocation. Clin Radiol 51:737-739

65. Neustadter J, Raikin SM, Nazarian LN (2004) Dynamic sonographic evaluation of peroneal tendon subluxation. AJR 183:985-988

66. Bianchi S, Martinoli C, Gaignot C et al (2005) Ultrasound of the ankle: anatomy of the tendons, bursae, and ligaments. Semin Musculoskelet Radiol 9:243-259

67. Chau CL, Griffith JF (2005) Musculoskeletal infections: ultrasound appearances. Clin Radiol 60:149-159

68. Bureau NJ, Chhem RK, Cardinal E (1999) Musculoskeletal infections: US manifestations.Radiographics 19:1585-1592

69. Okayama A, Futani H, Kyo F et al (2003) Usefulness of ultrasonography for early recurrent myositis ossificans. J Orthop Sci 8:239-242

70. Park A, Lehnerdt G, Lautermann J (2006) Myositis of the sternocleidomastoid muscle as a result of arthritis of the sternoclavicular joint. Laryngorhinootologie. Epub ahead of print

71. De Marchi A, De Petro P, Linari A et al (2002) Preliminary experience in the study of soft tissue superficial masses. Color-Doppler US and wash-in and wash-out curves with contrast media compared to histological result. Radiol Med 104:451-458

72. De Marchi A, De Petro P, Faletti C et al (2003) Echocolor power Doppler with contrast medium to evaluate vascularization in lesions of the soft tissues of the limbs. Chir Organi Mov 88:225-231

73. Melis M, Marongiu L, Scintu F et al (2002) Primary hydatid cysts of psoas muscle. ANZ J Surg 72:443-445

74. Peetrons P (2002) Ultrasound of muscles. Eur Radiol 12:35-43

75. Newman JS, Adler RS, Bude RO, Rubin JM (1994) Detection of soft-tissue hyperemia: value of power Doppler sonography. AJR 163:385-389

76. Krix M, Weber MA, Krakowski-Roosen H et al (2005) Assessment of skeletal muscle perfusion using contrast-enhanced ultrasonography. J Ultrasound Med 24:431-441

77. Hammer HB, Hovden IA, Haavardsholm EA et al (2005) Ultrasonography shows increased cross-sectional area of the median nerve in patients with arthritis and carpal tunnel syndrome. Rheumatology (in press)

78. Beekman R, Visser LH (2004) High-resolution sonography of the peripheral nervous system: a review of the literature. Eur J Neurology 11:305-314

79. Ziswiler HR, Reichenbach S, Vögelin E et al (2005) Diagnostic value of sonography in patients with suspected carpal tunnel syndrome: a prospective study. Arthritis Rheum 52:304-311

80. Redd RA, Peters VJ, Emery SF et al (1989) Morton neuroma: sonographic evaluation. Radiology 171:415-417

81. Read JW, Noakes JB, Kerr D et al (1999) Morton's metatarsalgia: sonographic findings and correlated histopathology. Foot Ankle Int 20:153-161

82. Sobiesk GA, Wertheimer SJ, Schulz R et al (1997) Sonographic evaluation of interdigital neuromas. J Foot Ankle Surg 36:364-366

83. Quinn TJ, Jacobson JA, Craig JG, van Holsbeeck MT (2000) Sonography of Morton's neuromas. AJR 174:1723-1728

84. Batz R, Sofka CM, Adler RS et al (2006) Dermatomyositis and calcific myonecrosis in the leg: ultrasound as an aid in management. Skeletal Radiol 35:113-116

85. Gibbon WW (2004) Applications of ultrasound in arthritis. Semin Musculoskelet Radiol 8:313-328

86. Inampudi P, Jacobson JA, Fessell DP et al (2004) Soft-tissue lipomas: accuracy of sonography in diagnosis with pathologic correlation. Radiology 233:763-767

87. Griffith JF, Wong TY, Wong SM et al (2002) Sonography of plantar fibromatosis. AJR 179:1167-1172

88. Teefey SA, Middleton WD, Boyer MI (2000) Sonography of the hand and wrist. Semin Ultrasound CT MR 21:192-204

Chapter 5

Pathological findings in rheumatic diseases

The ability of US to make an accurate evaluation of soft tissue involvement in a wide range of diseases of the locomotor system has led to its increasing widespread use in the field of rheumatology [1-10]. Significant technological progress has been made over the last few years, generating ever more sophisticated and reliable ultrasound machinery. The high resolution is now such that real *in vivo* histological examination is now possible. The main reason for the relative lack of wide diffusion of its use amongst rheumatologists is that a long training period is necessary in order to acquire full operator independence.

Initially, the use of US in rheumatology was limited to the identification of large collections of synovial fluid (popliteal cysts, bursitis) [11]. These collections can be easily identified even with 'first generation' US equipment that uses probes with frequencies between 3.5 and 5 MHz. These are, however, inappropriate for the study of superficial soft tissues. With the advent of the 'second generation' US machines, with 7.5 MHz linear probes, US can now explore larger joints. Clinical practice now includes the study of the shoulder, hip and knee has proven useful in the examination of large tendons (Achilles, long head of biceps and patellar tendon).

The potential applications of US in rheumatology have been further increased with the dawn of the 'third generation' US machines, equipped with very high-frequency probes (> 10 MHz). These can reach a spatial resolution of less than a tenth of a millimeter and make it possible to study the finest details of the smaller joints and hand tendons which are involved early on in chronic arthritis.

5.1 Osteoarthritis

Several sonographic abnormalities may be observed in patients with osteoarthritis. These include changes within cartilage, joint cavity widening resulting from fluid collection with or without synovial proliferation, and osteophytes [12-14].

Changes within cartilage

Loss of the thin, sharp contour of the superficial margin of the cartilaginous layer is one of the early features of osteoarthritis. US is exquisitely sensitive in detecting structural changes within different tissues and can reveal fibrillation and cleft formation in osteoarthritis (Fig. 5.1) [15].

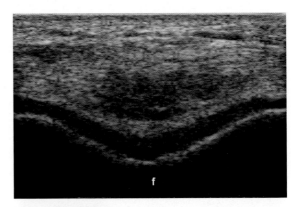

Fig. 5.1

Osteoarthritis. Supra-patellar transverse scan with knee in maximal flexion shows loss of the normal clarity of cartilage layer together with blurring of the superficial margin of the femoral condylar cartilage. *f* = femur

Increased echogenicity with patchy or diffuse loss of clarity may be seen even in patients without any other findings to indicate damage to the cartilage structure. These changes would seem to reflect structural alterations such as fibrillation of cartilage and cleft formation [13]. Particular attention should be paid to distinguish these early findings in osteoarthritis from artifacts caused by inaccurate setting (gain level) or probe position [16].

A slight increase in cartilage thickness caused by inflammatory edema in the early phases of osteoarthritis has been noted [13]. Variable narrowing of the cartilaginous layer is detectable in patients at a more advanced stage of the disease. Cartilage thinning may be focal, or extend along the entire cartilaginous layer (Fig. 5.2).

US measurement of femoral condyle articular cartilage thickness could be of practical benefit for an early diagnosis of osteoarthritis. Accurate quantification of cartilage thickness cannot always be obtained in patients with advanced osteoarthritis because of poor visualization of the cartilage-synovial space interface. Complete cartilage loss can be observed in advanced disease (Fig. 5.3) [12, 13, 17].

Supra-patellar scanning of weight-bearing areas can be difficult in patients with advanced osteoarthritis and/or painful knee, resulting in limited maximal active flexion [15-18]. Diagnostic accuracy in the detection and grading of cartilage abnormalities should be the subject of further research. The knee and the metacarpophalangeal joints are the locations in which US can best demonstrate the various evolutionary phases of cartilage involvement in osteoarthritis.

The articular cartilage of the metacarpal head can be evaluated by longitudinal and transverse dorsal scans, with the metacarpophalangeal joint held in maximal active flexion. Standard longitudinal dorsal and volar scans may also be useful.

Proximal and distal interphalangeal joints are generally evaluated by means of longitudinal and transverse dorsal scans with the finger in a neutral position. US with high frequency probes allows for an in-depth study of these joints, even if only a limited portion of the cartilage can be explored, due to the acoustic barriers (Fig. 5.4 a, b, c)

Joint effusion

Small to moderate joint effusions are commonly found in patients with osteoarthritis (Figs. 5.5, 5.6, 5.7). Minimal fluid collections that may be missed on clinical examination are easily detected by US. Synovial fluid is usually anechoic. Non-homogeneous echogenicity of synovial fluid and/or echogenic spots with or without acoustic shadowing can be generated by proteinaceous material, cartilage fragments, crystal aggregates and calcified loose bodies.

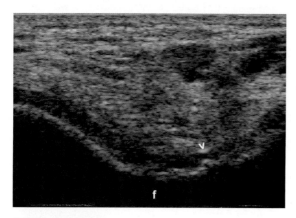

Fig. 5.2

Osteoarthritis. Supra-patellar transverse scan with knee in maximal flexion demonstrates focal cartilage thinning (*arrowhead*) and marked irregularity of the subchondral bone. *f* = femur

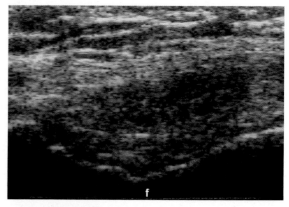

Fig. 5.3

Osteoarthritis. Supra-patellar transverse scan with knee in maximal flexion shows complete loss of cartilage. *f* = femur

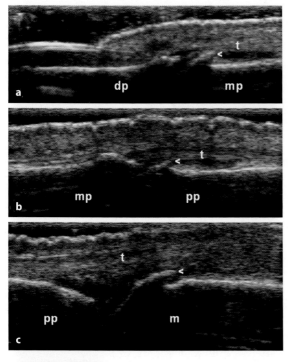

Fig. 5.4 a-c

Osteoarthritis. Index finger of the dominant hand. Dorsal longitudinal views. **a** Distal interphalangeal joint. **b** Proximal interphalangeal joint. **c** Metacarpophalangeal joint. *dp* = distal phalanx; *mp* = middle phalanx; *pp* = proximal phalanx; *m* = metacarpal bone; *t* = extensor tendon; *arrowhead* = osteophyte

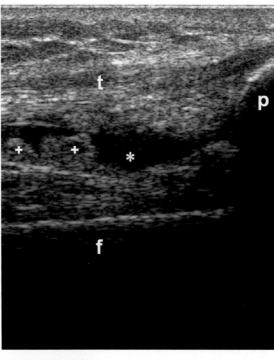

Fig. 5.5

Osteoarthritis. Supra-patellar longitudinal US scan showing widening of the supra-patellar pouch due to synovial fluid (*) and proliferation (+). *f* = femur; *p* = upper pole of the patella; *t* = quadriceps tendon

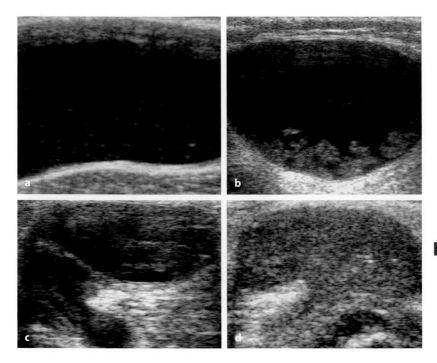

Fig. 5.6 a-d

Osteoarthritis of the knee. Different US features of popliteal cysts. **a** Anechoic with floating echogenic spots. **b** Areas of synovial proliferation. **c** Septa and areas of synovial proliferation. **d** Completely filled by synovial proliferation

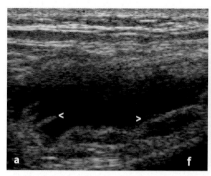 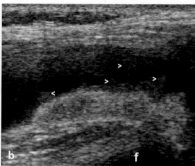

Fig. 5.7 a, b

Osteoarthritis of the knee. Lateral longitudinal views of the suprapatellar pouch showing different aspects of synovial proliferation (*arrowheads*). *f* = femur

Fine particulate debris floating in the synovial fluid is generally observed after long-standing or repeated joint effusions or after intra-articular corticosteroid administration.

In patients with asymptomatic Heberden's nodes, there is usually no detectable joint space widening. Conversely, symptomatic joint involvement is frequently associated with variable capsular distension (Fig. 5.8 a, b).

Popliteal cysts are a frequent finding in patients with knee osteoarthritis (Fig. 5.6 a-d). US provides structural details about the content of the cyst, its communication with the joint space and possible compression of adjacent vascular structures. Both the size and shape of cysts vary widely, ranging from small (<1 cm) to giant, multi-loculated entities.

Synovial proliferation

Synovial proliferation in osteoarthritis may display US features similar to those observed in patients with chronic inflammatory arthritis but without the invasive properties of rheumatoid pannus (Fig. 5.7 a, b). Thickened, edematous synovium is frequently observed in more severe disease and in patients with recurrent effusions.

Osteophytes

Osteophytes are easily detected as irregularities of the bone contour. The skyline view of an osteoarthritic joint is characteristic and correlates with conventional radiographic changes (Fig. 5.9 a, b).

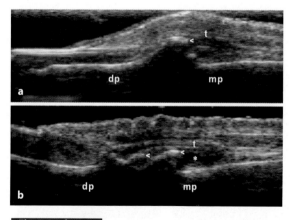

Fig. 5.8 a, b

Heberden's nodes. Longitudinal dorsal US scan. **a** Symptomatic joint. Dorsal subluxation of the distal phalanx with no evidence of joint inflammation. **b** Symptomatic joint. Joint effusion (*) and osteophytes (*arrowheads*). *dp* = distal phalanx; *mp* = middle phalanx; *t* = extensor tendon; *arrowhead* = osteophyte

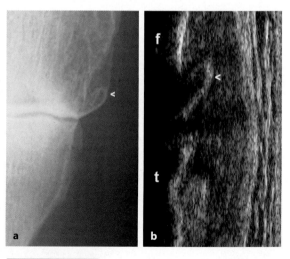

Fig. 5.9 a, b

Osteophytes in knee osteoarthritis. **a** Conventional radiography. **b** Medial longitudinal US scan showing an osteophyte of the femoral condyle (*arrowhead*). *f* = femur; *t* = tibia

Erosive osteoarthritis

Sonographic findings in patients with erosive osteoarthritis usually combine the aspects of both osteoarthritis (osteophytes and subluxation of the articular surfaces) and inflammatory involvement (joint space widening and intra-articular power Doppler signal) (Fig. 5.10 a, b) [19, 20].

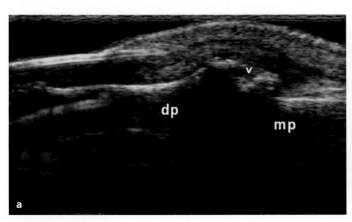
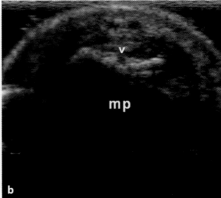

Fig. 5.10 a, b

Erosive osteoarthritis of the distal interphalangeal joint. The arrowhead indicates a bone erosion at the head of the middle phalanx depicted both on longitudinal (**a**) and transverse (**b**) dorsal sonograms. *dp* = distal phalanx; *mp* = middle phalanx

5.2 Rheumatoid arthritis

US in patients with rheumatoid arthritis demonstrates a wide range of anomalies [21-31]. It provides detailed information on the quantity and characteristics of the fluid collection, the presence of synovial proliferation and the integrity of articular cartilage and subchondral bone.

Joint effusion

Distension of the joint capsule and the increase in volume of synovial fluid are the most common initial US findings. In these embryonic stages of the disease the synovitis is prevalently exudative and the content of the joint space is characterized by its homogenous anechogenicity (Fig. 5.11).

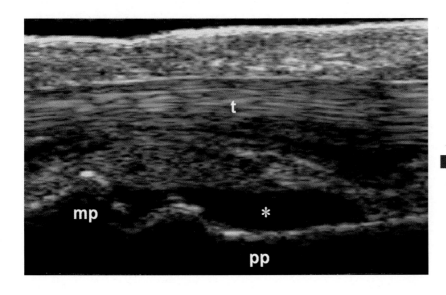

Fig. 5.11

Early rheumatoid arthritis. Exudative synovitis of the proximal interphalangeal joint of the dominant hand. Longitudinal volar scan depicting anechoic joint cavity widening (*). *mp* = middle phalanx; *pp* = proximal phalanx; *t* = extensor tendon

US makes it possible to document the presence of even minimal distension of the joint capsule and of intra and peri-articular synovial fluid collection (synovial cysts, bursitis).

Synovial proliferation

Proliferation of the synovial membrane appears as hypoechoic thickening of the 'internal capsular wall' which can be either homogenous or adopt various conformations (villous, polypoid, or bushy appearance) (Fig. 5.12).

These appearances can be documented even in early stages of the disease. Synovial hypertrophy should be differentiated from the accumulation of proteinaceous material or leukocytes that are mildly echogenic or finely granular with a cloudy appearance that changes upon palpation with the probe over the skin surface. The identification of synovial proliferation in finger joints together with the evaluation of pannus perfusion using power Doppler has heralded the search for pre-erosive changes in rheumatoid arthritis (Fig. 5.13). Highly vascularized synovial pannus can predict radiologographic damage in rheumatoid arthritis and therefore the presence of synovial proliferation represents an important element in the classification of early arthritis.

Bone erosions

Over the last few years, several studies in rheumatoid arthritis have confirmed that ultrasonography permits accurate and detailed analysis of the anatomical changes induced by the inflammatory process and is more sensitive than conventional X-rays for the detection of bone erosions [24-26].

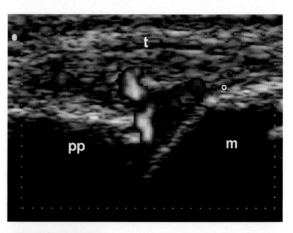

Fig. 5.13

Rheumatoid arthritis. Proliferative synovitis of the second metacarpophalangeal joint of the dominant hand. Longitudinal dorsal scan depicting hyperperfused areas of synovial hypertrophy invading the cartilage layer of the metacarpal head (°). *pp* = proximal phalanx; *m* = metacarpal bone; *t* = extensor tendon

This higher sensitivity in the detection of erosions depends both on the high spatial resolution of the high-frequency transducers and on the possibility of carrying out multiplanar examination (Fig. 5.14 a-d).

Bone erosions are viewed on US as an interruption of the sharp hyperechoic bone profile with the wall and the floor, in most cases filled by hyperperfused synovial pannus.

At the level of the metacarpophalangeal joints, US can identify a number of erosions much more frequently than conventional X-ray in patients with early rheumatoid arthritis [26]. The radial aspect of the second metacarpal head and the lateral aspect of the fifth metatarsal head are the anatomical locations where 'micro-erosions' in 'early arthritis' can

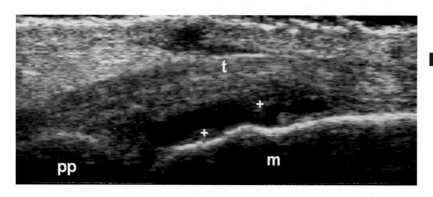

Fig. 5.12

Rheumatoid arthritis. Proliferative synovitis of the second metacarpophalangeal joint of the dominant hand. Longitudinal dorsal scan detecting very small areas (less than 1 mm in size) of synovial proliferation (+). *pp* = proximal phalanx; *m* = metacarpal bone; *t* = extensor tendon

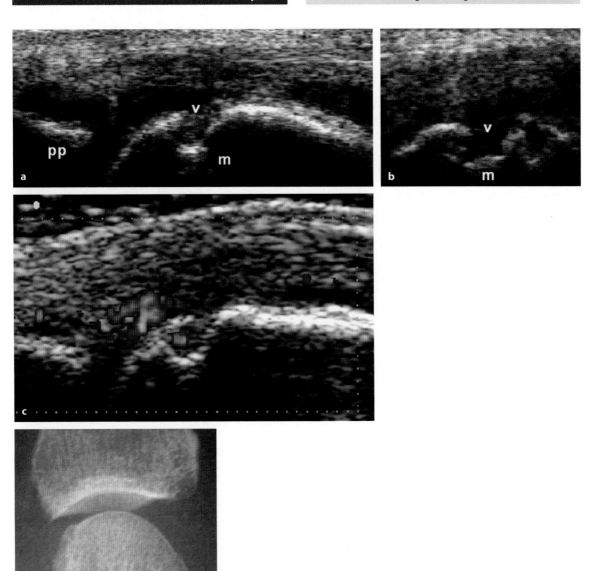

Fig. 5.14 a-d

Rheumatoid arthritis. Proliferative synovitis of the second metacarpophalangeal joint of the dominant hand. Dorsal longitudinal (**a**) and transverse (**b**) scans showing clear signs of synovial proliferation and bone erosion of the metacarpal head (*arrowhead*). **c** Intra-articular power Doppler signal. **d** Conventional radiography. *pp* = proximal phalanx; *m* = metacarpal bone

be recognized [25]. In both areas longitudinal scans should be integrated with transverse scans both in order to confirm the findings and to ensure exploration of a greater surface area of the bone profiles (Figs. 5.14, 5.15).

In patients with rheumatoid arthritis the fifth metatarsophalangeal joint is an early target for aggressive synovitis. At this level, US can detect even minimal erosions which are often missed by conventional X-ray.

Conventional morphological study should always be integrated with power Doppler study, when seeking to confirm synovitis in an active phase (Fig. 5.16 a-d) [29, 31-35].

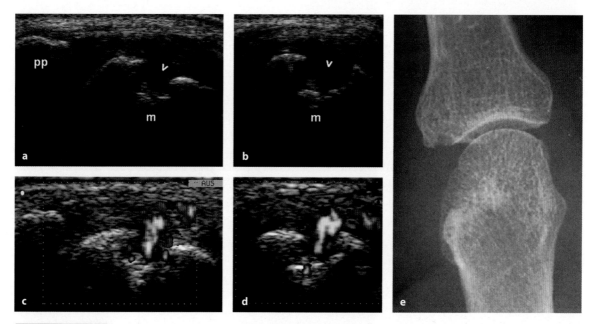

Fig. 5.15 a-e

Rheumatoid arthritis. Proliferative synovitis of the second metacarpophalangeal joint of the dominant hand. Lateral (on the radial aspect of the joint) longitudinal (**a**) and transverse (**b**) scans showing a large erosion (*arrowhead*) (maximal distance between the edges of the erosion: 4 mm). **c, d** Using the same scanning planes, power Doppler revealed hyperperfused pannus within the bone erosion. **e** Conventional radiography. *pp* = proximal phalanx; *m* = metacarpal bone

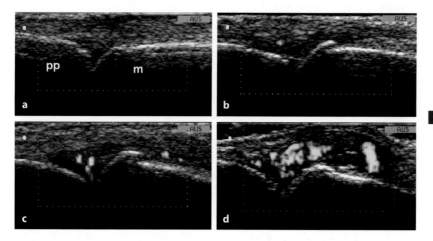

Fig. 5.16 a-d

Rheumatoid arthritis. Semi-quantitative scoring system for intra-articular power Doppler signal. **a** Grade 0; no intra-articular signal. **b** Grade 1; single intra-articular signal. **c** Grade 2; confluent intra-articular signals. **d** Grade 3; huge amount of intra-articular signals

Tendon involvement

US is particularly useful in the study of tendon involvement in early rheumatoid arthritis, which often accompanies and in some cases precedes evidence of the disease at joint level. The range of tendon change in rheumatoid arthritis is wide and includes distension of the tendon sheath, loss of 'fibrillar' echotexture, loss of definition of tendon margins and the partial or complete loss of tendon continuity [36].

US is of very important practical value in the evaluation of finger tendons. Tendon sheath widening is the hallmark of early tendon involvement in rheumatoid arthritis and other conditions characterized by synovial inflammation. Several US patterns of tendon sheath widening can be characterized by the extent of the widening, amount of syn-

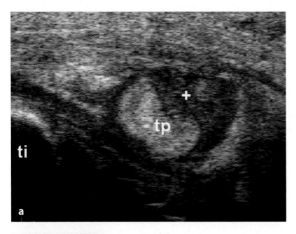 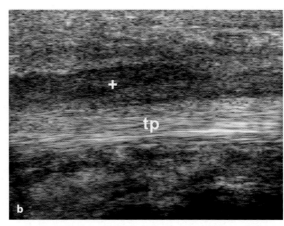

Fig. 5.17 a, b

Rheumatoid arthritis. Proliferative tenosynovitis of the tibialis posterior tendon (*tp*). Transverse (**a**) and longitudinal (**b**) scans showing a tendon sheath filled with pannus (+). ti = tibia

ovial fluid within the sheath, profile of the tendon sheath, echogenicity of the sheath content and the presence of synovial hypertrophy.

The amount of synovial fluid within a widened tendon sheath may vary considerably, ranging from minimal homogeneous widening (difficult to detect if the pressure of the transducer is too high) to dramatic, balloon-like distension. There is no direct relationship between the extent of tendon sheath widening and clinical symptoms.

The profile of a widened tendon sheath can be regular or extremely non-homogeneous with saccular or aneurysmal appearance, especially in chronic tenosynovitis. The appearance of sheath content is characteristically anechoic in patients with acute tenosynovitis. Conversely, if synovial fluid is rich in proteinaceous material or has an elevated cellular content, a variable degree of soft echoes can be detected. The use of very high frequency transducers allows for the detection of synovial hypertrophy which appears as an irregular thickening of the synovial layer and/or bushy or villous vegetations (Fig. 5.17 a, b) [22].

Analysis of tendon echotexture is one of the fundamental aims of US examination. Circumscribed abnormalities of the homogenous distribution of the intratendinous connective fibers are the unequivocal expression of anatomical damage mediated by the process of chronic inflammation. In the early phases of inflammation the morphological picture is that of 'tendon erosion' that can precede a more extended 'loss of substance' and evolve into a partial or complete tendon tear (Fig. 5.18 a-e).

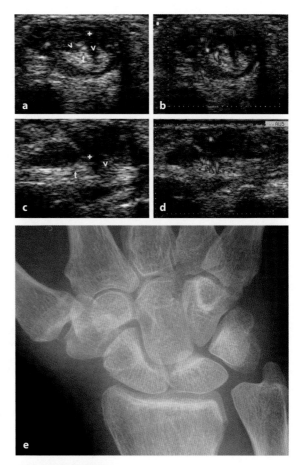

Fig. 5.18 a-e

Rheumatoid arthritis. Wrist pain. Lateral transverse (**a, b**) and longitudinal (**c, d**) scans showing active proliferative tenosynovitis of the extensor carpi ulnaris tendon (*t*) with partial tendon rupture (*arrowheads*). **e** Conventional radiography

Where 'tendon erosion' is suspected, this diagnosis should always be confirmed by dynamic investigation and comparison with images taken on longitudinal and transverse scans. This is in order to exclude the possibility of artifacts due to altered inclination of the probe rather than a real anatomical alteration. It may be difficult to differentiate between partial tendon tear and tendon degeneration. The term 'intrasubstance abnormality' or 'intrasubstance tear' is often used to describe irregular areas of very low echogenicity within the tendon. More commonly, partial tendon tears appear clearest on transverse views, but the possibility of an artifact should always be kept in mind and the suspicion of a tendon tear on a single field of observation must be verified along contiguous slices with the US beam held perfectly perpendicular to the tendon (Figs. 5.19, 5.20).

Inadequate transducer positioning is the most frequent source of false diagnosis of tendon tear. Complete tendon tear is easily detectable especially if tendons with synovial sheaths are involved (empty sheath sign). The edges of the torn tendon are frequently retracted and curled up.

Power Doppler studies make it possible to document hyperemia associated with the phases of active inflammation, also at the level of the tendon.

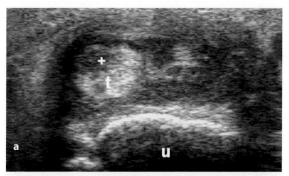
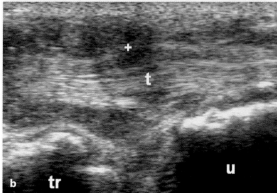

Fig. 5.19 a, b

Rheumatoid arthritis. Wrist pain. Lateral transverse (**a**) and longitudinal (**b**) scans showing proliferative tenosynovitis of the extensor carpi ulnaris tendon (*t*) with pannus (+) invading the tendon texture (*arrowheads*). *u* = ulna; *tr* = triquetrum

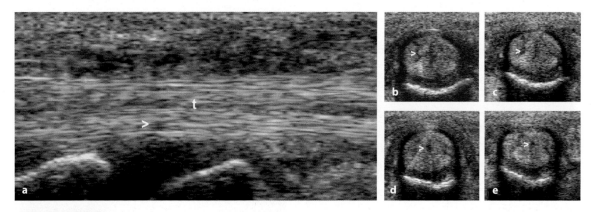

Fig. 5.20 a-e

Rheumatoid arthritis. Finger flexor tendons. Tenosynovitis and tendon tears. Longitudinal (**a**) and cross-sectional (**b-e**) volar scanning of the finger flexor tendons (*t*) at the level of the metacarpophalangeal joint. Tendon tears appear as small anechoic areas (less than 1 millimeter) within tendon echotexture (*arrowheads*)

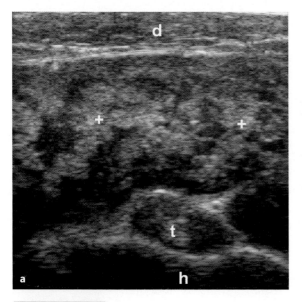
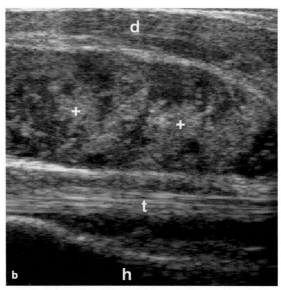

Fig. 5.21 a, b

Rheumatoid arthritis. Shoulder pain. Transverse (**a**) and longitudinal (**b**) anterior scans at the bicipital groove. Proliferative subdeltoid bursitis and tenosynovitis of the long head of biceps tendon (*t*). *h* = humerus; *d* = deltoid

Bursitis

Finally, ultrasonography allows clear documentation of involvement of synovial bursae in rheumatoid arthritis. A significant increase in the volume of synovial fluid makes the bursa, which quite often contain signs of synovial hypertrophy, easily visible (Fig. 5.21).

5.3 Seronegative spondyloarthritis

The US imagery present in psoriatic arthritis is similar to that seen in rheumatoid arthritis.

Distal interphalangeal involvement can be accurately documented with probes of frequencies greater than 10 MHz. Distension of the joint capsule is easily detected together with edema of the periarticular soft tissues (Fig. 5.22).

US can distinguish between soft tissue swelling and the presence of bony swelling in a Heberden node [19].

The 'sausage' finger, which is a common finding in psoriatic arthritis, is characterized by the following US features [37, 38]:
1. distension of the flexor sheath;
2. distension of the joint capsule of the proximal interphalangeal joints;
3. edema along the entire thickness of the soft tissues.

The presence of tenosynovitis has been confirmed frequently in the 'sausage' finger, but in some cases may be entirely absent (Fig. 5.23).

Involvement of tendons without a synovial sheath (Achilles tendon, patellar tendon), together with pathology located at the enthesis and aponeurosis, can have a wide range of characteristic US features [39–45]. Achilles tendonitis is characterized by thickening of the tendon that can adopt a fusiform appearance and show hypoechogenicity secondary to edema. In addition, peritendinitis (hypoechogenicity at the level of the peritenon) and edema of soft tissues can co-exist (Fig. 5.24). The detection of distension of the deep retrocalcaneal bursa is particularly common.

Enthesitis can be depicted in all stages of its evolution by US. In the early stages, the bone profile shows no significant change whilst the area of the enthesis and the adjacent portion of the tendon show hypoechogenicity. In more advanced phases, discontinuity of the bone profile at the point of insertion is more clearly depicted and can evolve into wide areas of re-absorption (Fig. 5.25).

As enthesitis advances even further, enthesophytes can be identified with a characteristic posterior acoustic cone of shadow. In the plantar fascia,

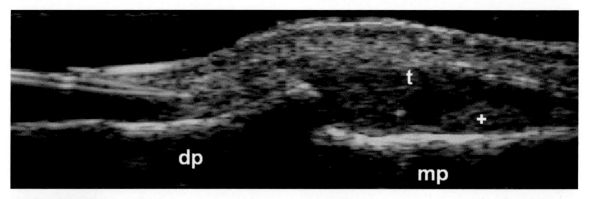

Fig. 5.22

Psoriatic arthritis. Distal interphalangeal joint. Dorsal longitudinal scan showing joint cavity widening and clear signs of synovial proliferation (+). *dp* = distal phalanx; *mp* = middle phalanx; *t* = extensor tendon

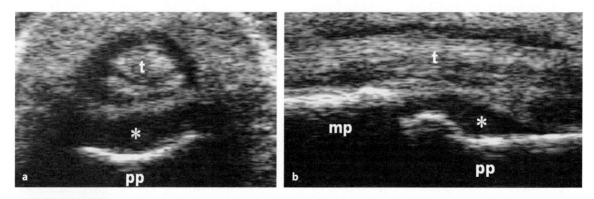

Fig. 5.23 a, b

Psoriatic arthritis. Sausage finger. Proximal interphalangeal joint. Volar transverse (**a**) and longitudinal (**b**) scans showing both tendon sheath and joint cavity widening. *mp* = middle phalanx; *pp* = proximal phalanx; *t* = flexor tendons; * = synovial fluid

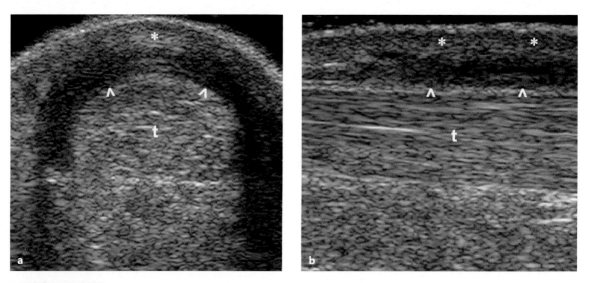

Fig. 5.24 a, b

Psoriatic arthritis. Peritendinitis of the Achilles tendon (*t*). Longitudinal (**a**) and transverse (**b**) scans showing thickened hypo-anechoic peritenon (*arrowheads*) with hypoechogenicity of the peritendinous soft tissues (*)

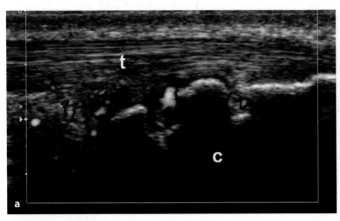 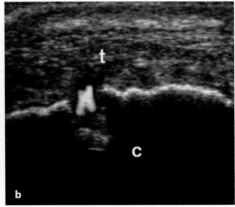

Fig. 5.25 a, b

Psoriatic arthritis. Achilles tendon (*t*). Erosive enthesitis. Longitudinal (**a**) and transverse (**b**) scans showing power Doppler signal within the calcaneal bone erosions. *c* = calcaneal bone

US can detect changes in fascial thickness, and in the peri-fascial adipose tissue which becomes hypoechogenic with a characteristic 'muff-like' appearance best seen on transverse scans.

Ultrasound examination of patients with hyperalgesic fascia is particularly useful during treatment when correct positioning of the needle to deliver local therapy can be confirmed.

Psoriatic involvement of the distal interphalangeal joints can be demonstrated with ultrasonography and features include joint space widening mainly on the longitudinal dorsal scan. The longitudinal volar scan confirms joint space widening together with any flexor tendon involvement which can be prominent.

5.4 Crystal-related arthropathies

Crystal-related arthropathies are a group of disorders in which minerals are deposited in musculoskeletal tissues, resulting in further pathological changes.

Both monosodium urate and calcium pyrophosphate dihydrate crystal aggregates can be clearly seen by ultrasonography in different anatomical areas and tissues. The spectrum of sonographic appearance of monosodium urate aggregation can vary from homogeneously punctuate (urate sand) to sharply defined hyperechoic densities of variable dimensions and eventually to dense tophaceous material that is impermeable to the ultrasound beam (Fig. 5.26).

The conformation and anatomical location of the crystal aggregates in pyrophosphate arthropathy are the main elements which help distinguish them from other crystalline arthropathies. The ability of ultrasonography to detect pyrophosphate crystals in joints with aspirated synovial fluid containing pyrophosphate crystals has been investigated with excellent results. Similar work has yet to be done in the setting of gout. The ease with which even minimal crystalline aggregates in pyrophosphate arthropathy and gout are visualized make ultrasonography a very promising tool to aid diagnosis. This is particularly pertinent in

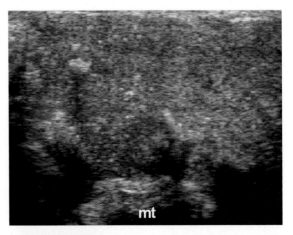

Fig. 5.26

Gout of the first metatarsophalangeal joint. Transverse lateral view depicting "urate sand". *mt* = metatarsal head

the setting of acute inflammatory arthritis when other imaging modalities may be negative or unavailable. Future research into crystalline arthropathies should employ US, particularly to investigate the link between pyrophosphate arthropathy and osteoarthritis and in the potential monitoring of therapy for gout.

Gout

In patients with acute gout, US examination of the first metatarsophalangeal joint reveals joint space widening due to the presence of variable amounts of fluid and within it monosodium urate crystals, which appear as irregular floating echoic spots (Fig. 5.27) [1, 46].

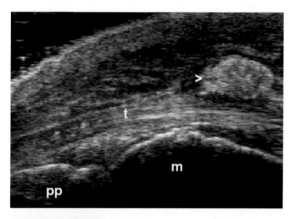

Fig. 5.27

Tophaceous gout. Longitudinal dorsal US scan of the first metatarsophalangeal joint showing "soft" tophus (*arrowhead*). The echotexture has an inhomogeneously echoic background with hyperechoic densities that do not generate posterior acoustic shadows. *mt* = metatarsal head; *pp* = proximal phalanx; *t* = extensor tendon

Fluid collections in patients with acute episodes of gout can show different sonographic patterns, ranging from homogeneous anechogenicity of the synovial fluid to aggregates of variable shape and echogenicity. Following sono-palpation (gentle pressure applied by the probe to the skin surface) of the joint being examined, these aggregates can be seen to float within the joint cavity giving rise to a 'snow-storm' appearance.

Tophaceous deposits may show a differing degree of reflectivity according to the level of compaction of the deposits. These vary from soft tophi, with typically varying echogenicity that are soft to palpation, to hard tophi that contain monosodium urate deposits generating a hyperechoic band and acoustic shadow and which are harder in consistency to palpation (Fig. 5.28) [19].

Intra-articular bone erosions frequently occur in patients with chronic gout. They are in some ways similar to those seen in rheumatoid arthritis, but tend to be deeper and more destructive. Extra-articular interruption of the bone profile due to intra-osseous tophi is easily detectable when the tophus is less compact and permits the passage of the ultrasound beam onto the bone surface.

The deposition of monosodium urate crystals within tendons can be variable depending on the size of the aggregates and on disease duration [47]. Micro-deposits, which can be observed in asymptomatic patients, appear as predominantly ovoid shaped hyperechoic densities.

These deposits maintain their high degree of reflectivity, even in situations where power and gain settings are minimized. The ensuing inflammatory response incited by these deposits generates a small hypoechoic 'halo' and sono-palpation of these areas can induce exquisite localized pain. The normal fibrillar echotexture of tendons can be

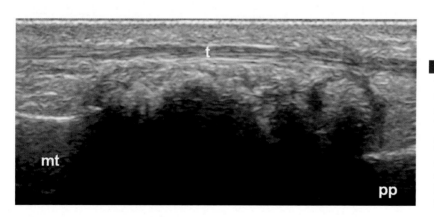

Fig. 5.28

Tophaceous gout. Longitudinal dorsal US scan of the first metatarsophalangeal joint showing "hard" tophus. The bone profile of the joint cannot be visualized due to the presence of extensive urate deposition obstructing the path of the US beam. *mt* = metatarsal head; *pp* = proximal phalanx; *t* = extensor tendon

completely deranged by the presence of intra-tendinous tophus formation, which appears as hypoechoic material with the occasional presence of hyperechoic spots. Long-standing intra-tendinous tophus appears as hyperechoic bands that may generate an acoustic shadow according to their size and density.

Pyrophosphate arthropathy

Crystalline deposits in pyrophosphate arthropathy within hyaline and/or meniscal cartilage appear as a homogenously echogenic band that in most cases does not generate a posterior acoustic shadow [48-51]. This generates the characteristic 'double bordered' appearance that is very similar to that seen on conventional X-ray (Fig. 5.29).

This phenomenon can be explained by the irregular distribution of the crystals along the cartilage surface, which makes it impossible for a homogenous barrier to echo transmission to form.

In patients with acute synovitis fine hyperechoic spots can be seen within the synovial fluid. These anomalies, which can be found almost exclusively in patients with chondrocalcinosis confirmed on synovial liquid microscopy, are assumed to represent pyrophosphate crystal aggregates.

The concentration and the dimensions of these aggregates may be particularly conspicuous in patients with dense and whitish synovial liquid (Fig. 5.30).

Echogenic aggregates are also seen in pyrophosphate arthropathy. These are typically uniformly rounded in shape, with a sharply-defined outer profile. They can be demonstrated in various anatomical areas including the knee and wrist joints, popliteal cysts and sub-deltoid bursae. Crystal aggregates should be distinguished from joint debris and proteinaceous material floating within

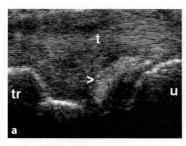
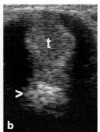
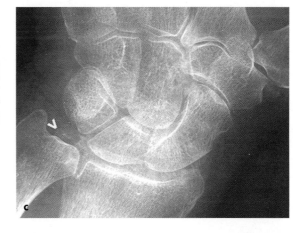

Fig. 5.29 a-c

Pyrophosphate arthropathy. Wrist joint. Longitudinal (**a**) and transverse (**b**) views. **c** X-ray. Calcification of the triangular ligament of the carpus (*arrowheads*). *t* = extensor ulnaris carpi tendon; *u* = ulna; *tr* = triquetrum

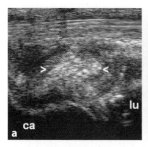
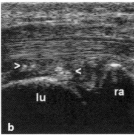
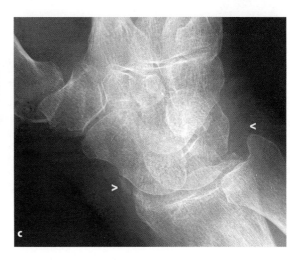

Fig. 5.30 a-c

Pyrophosphate arthropathy. Dorsal (**a**) and volar (**b**) longitudinal views of the wrist reveal large crystal deposits (*arrowheads*). **c** X-ray. *ca* = capitate bone; *lu* = lunate bone; *ra* = radius

the joint cavity by demonstrating the reflectivity of the crystals present through adjustment of the ultrasound setting to a low level of power and gain.

Calcification of tendons in pyrophosphate arthropathy is typically linear, extensive and may generate an acoustic shadow. They must be distinguished from apatite deposits which are generally more discreet and nummular in conformation.

Apatite deposition disease

Calcific periarthritis is the main apatite-related condition. Calcium deposits are clearly detected because of their high reflectivity and generation of an acoustic shadow. Calcium deposits are, however, not always associated with posterior acoustic shadow and are connected to the degree of com-

paction of the crystalline aggregates (Fig. 5.31). Slurry calcifications have a nearly liquid consistency and can be aspirated. Their size, shape and location can vary significantly. In patients with acute inflammatory symptoms soft tissues surrounding the calcium deposits may show a hypoechoic pattern due to edema. Increased power Doppler signal is a frequent finding. In clinically asymptomatic patients, single or multiple calcifications can often be observed.

With the dawn of US, there has been a significant upturn in the diagnosis of 'painful shoulder' [52-56]. US examination accurately documents the anatomical target of the variants of periarthropathy.

In tenosynovitis of the long head of the biceps tendon, the most characteristic US finding is distension of the tendon sheath (Fig. 5.32).

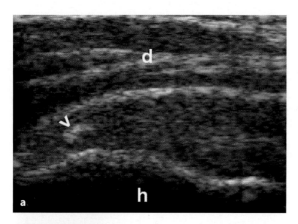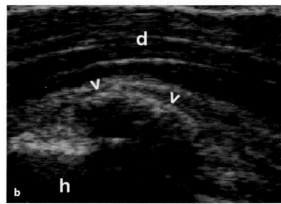

Fig. 5.31 a, b

Apatite deposition disease of the shoulder. Longitudinal scan (**a, b**) of the supraspinatus tendon. Intratendinous calcification without (**a**) and with (**b**) posterior acoustic shadow (*arrowhead*). *d* = deltoid; *h* = humerus

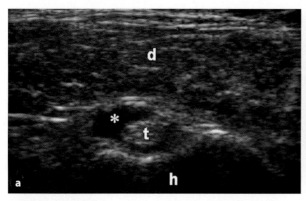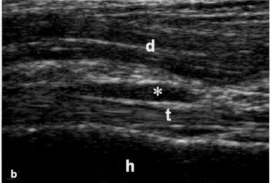

Fig. 5.32 a, b

Exudative tenosynovitis in shoulder pain. Transverse (**a**) and longitudinal (**b**) anterior scans at the bicipital groove. Mild anechoic tendon sheath widening (***). *h* = humerus; *t* = long biceps tendon; *d* = deltoid

In lesions of the rotator cuff, US makes it possible to document a wide range of changes, which include thinning of the supraspinatus tendon, deposition of hydroxyapatite crystal aggregates and partial or complete tendon tears (Fig. 5.33) [55, 56].

Subacromial-deltoid bursitis is fairly easily detected due to the generally conspicuous fluid collection that separates the walls. All patients with acute 'painful shoulder' must be examined with US methodically given the possibility that there may be more than one anomaly within the same individual.

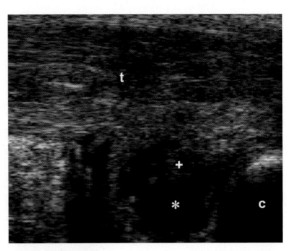

Fig. 5.34

Chronic tendinopathy of the Achilles tendon (*t*) in a patient with heterozygous familial hypercholesterolemia. Longitudinal US scan showing irregular fusiform thickening of the tendon, loss of the normal fibrillar echotexture, multiple areas of hypoechogenicity due to lipid infiltration and retrocalcaneal bursitis. *c* = calcaneal bone; * = synovial fluid; + = synovial proliferation

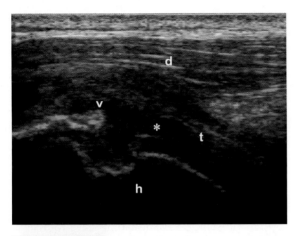

Fig. 5.33

Shoulder pain in patient with partial rupture of the supraspinatus tendon (*t*). Discontinuity of the tendon fibrils appearing as a hypoechoic area (*) with the same shape of the distal echo-free edge of the supraspinatus tendon (*arrowhead*). *h* = humerus; *d* = deltoid

5.5 Metabolic diseases

Tendon involvement is a prominent feature in patients with type II familial hypercholesterolemia. US is useful in establishing the diagnosis of heterozygous familial hypercholesterolemia in subjects with high levels of cholesterol and with no clinically evident xanthomata [57]. Tendon xanthomata appear as focal or confluent hypoechoic areas (Fig. 5.34).

The typical sonographic appearance of tendinosis is characterized by areas of altered echogenicity. Defects in tendon contour (blurring of the tendon margins) and loss of the normal fibrillar echotexture are frequent findings in patients with chronic tendinitis, post-traumatic tendinopathy, and in patients with metabolic disorders. Detection of intratendinous alteration of the normal fibrillar structure may be an important diagnostic clue to the presence of low mechanical resistance. Lack of homogeneity of tendon structure may range from focal aspects of fibrillar interruption to diffuse blurring of the tendon texture.

Intratendinous calcification is a frequent finding in patients with chronic inflammatory or degenerative tendinopathy and is frequently associated with endocrine and metabolic diseases (diabetes mellitus and familial hypercholesterolemia) (Fig. 5.35).

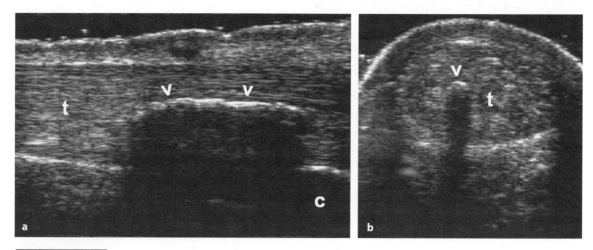

Calcific tendinopathy of the Achilles tendon (*t*). Longitudinal (**a**) and transverse (**b**) scans showing an intratendinous hyperechoic line (*arrowheads*) generating an acoustic shadow. *c* = calcaneal bone

5.6 Connective tissue diseases

Systemic lupus erythematosus

Synovitis is a frequent early finding in patients with systemic lupus erythematosus. Fluid collection with consequent joint cavity widening and increased power Doppler signal is the most characteristic sonographic feature [58]. Unlike rheumatoid arthritis, the ensuing synovitis is not characterized by the presence of bone erosions. Spontaneous or treatment-induced short term changes in US appearance of arthritis are frequently observed.

Systemic sclerosis

Very high frequency US probes (> 20 MHz) make it possible to study skin and subcutaneous involvement in patients with systemic sclerosis [59]. At present, US is showing great promise in this area of rheumatology. US findings in systemic sclerosis include soft tissue calcification and narrowing of the distance between phalangeal apex and skin surface at the distal phalanx (Fig. 5.36). Moreover, color and power Doppler may play a valuable role in the assessment of blood perfusion.

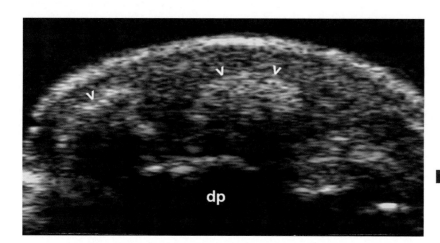

Calcinosis in systemic sclerosis. Longitudinal volar scan of the tip of the finger. *arrowheads* = calcification; *dp* = distal phalanx

5.7 Synovial osteochondromatosis

Primary synovial osteochondromatosis is an idiopathic metaplasia of the synovium, and may involve any synovial joint. This tumor-like condition is usually monoarticular and is rarely polyarticular. The disease is characterized by the presence of metaplastic chondroid islands confined to intrasynovial regions. Later on, cartilaginous foci spread and finally become calcified. Detachment of some calcified lobules gives rise to intra-articular loose bodies of various sizes. The affected joints do not appear inflamed; however, joint effusion may be occasionally present. The condition progresses slowly and can lead to secondary erosive and arthritic changes of joint bones.

The US appearance of synovial osteochondromatosis is characterized by numerous small echogenic foci. Most of these are associated with distal acoustic shadowing, corresponding to the conglomeration of calcified chondroid islands [16]. The synovium may be thickened.

US can suggest the presence of synovial osteochondromatosis, but is not definetively diagnostic. Therefore, conventional radiography is usually required to confirm the suspected diagnosis (Fig. 5.37).

Release of intra-articular loose bodies is not frequent. They appear as single or multiple echogenic foci with posterior acoustic shadowing, free-floating in the articular cavity when an effusion is present.

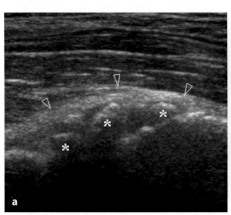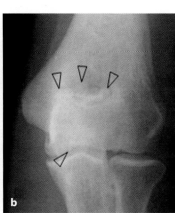

Fig. 5.37 a, b

Synovial osteochondromatosis of the elbow. **a** Longitudinal US scan of the anterior aspect of the elbow showing bulge and thickening of the capsular profile (*empty white arrowheads*). Multiple echogenic foci with posterior acoustic shadowing (*) lining synovial profile are evident. **b** Frontal radiograph in same patient showing several rounded opacities (*empty black arrowheads*), corresponding to calcified chondroid islands

5.8 Pigmented villonodular synovitis

Pigmented villonodular synovitis is a slow growing, benign synovial proliferative disorder that affects joints, bursae and tendon sheaths. Its etiology is controversial. The disease can present in three forms. First, the most common presentation affects the tendon sheaths – the so called giant cell tumor of the tendon sheaths – that appear as nodular tenosynovitis. It commonly occurs in the hands but has been identified in the foot as well. The typical feature in this form is the appearance of a painless mass on the finger. The other two forms of appearance are the localized form (nodular) and the diffuse form [60], which can be characterized by bursal and joint involvement. The disease is usually monoarticular and most commonly affects the knee, both in localized and diffuse presentation.

Initially, patients usually present with symptoms of mild discomfort and associated stiffness of the involved joint. Later on, pain and joint swelling may be evident.

The presenting US pattern in villonodular synovitis is non-specific. It usually appears as hypertrophied synovium, thickened and nodular, and relatively homogeneously hypoechoic. Power Doppler US demonstrates increased flow within the mass [61]. Tenosynovial involvement by the giant cell tumor most commonly appears as single hypoechoic nodule [16], which tends to surround and dislocate the tendons (Fig. 5.38).

This pathological condition, both in the articular and extra-articular form, may be associated with blood-stained effusion.

Later on, the synovial nodule can erode the adjacent bone.

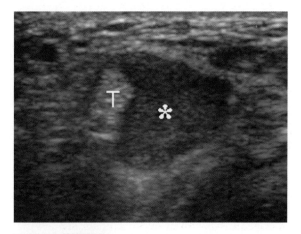

Fig. 5.38

Giant cell tumor of the hand. Transverse US scan of the palmar surface of the finger demonstrates a solid, relatively homogeneous hypoechoic mass (*), filling the tendon sheath. Tendons (T) are peripherally dislocated

5.9 Septic arthritis

Septic arthritis demonstrates great variability in US presentation, depending on patient age, etiological agent, evolutionary stage and affected joint. The US appearance can range from mild echogenic articular effusion to joint destruction (Fig. 5.39).

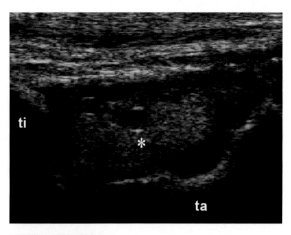

Fig. 5.39

Tibio-talar septic arthritis. Joint effusion appears inhomogeneously echogenic with turbid and sand-like appearance (*) suggestive of septic fluid collection. ti = tibia; ta = talus

When the diagnosis of septic arthritis is presumed, US may be mostly beneficial not only for a diagnostic confirmation, but also for therapeutic intervention. In fact, sonography is clearly highly sensitive in detecting joint effusions and may also guide a careful arthrocentesis, allowing drainage of minimal amounts of deep-seated septic fluid.

In infants and children particularly, septic arthritis can have potentially serious consequences and is considered a medical emergency. Prompt diagnosis is of paramount importance to avoid a disastrous outcome, which can lead to joint destruction when the therapy is delayed or inadequate.

Septic arthritis is relatively frequent in infancy, most commonly involving the hip joint. A classic presentation of septic arthritis is a sudden onset of the pain and joint discomfort, and the presence of clinical parameters proposed by Kocher (fever > 37.5°; erythrocyte sedimentation rate (ESR) > 40mm/hr; increase in serum white blood cell (WBC) count > 12.000/mm³). None of these are highly sensitive or specific for septic arthritis. Septic arthritis must always be excluded even in situations where the clinical presentation is atypical. In this way, US plays a primary role in differential diagnosis.

The US hallmarks of septic arthritis are articular effusion with inhomogeneous echogenicity, synovial thickening, and frequently synovial hypervascularity upon power Doppler US [62]. At the first evaluation, bone erosion may already be visualized (Fig. 5.40).

Transient synovitis in children can mimic septic arthritics. US examination shows evidence of joint effusion, which generally appears anechoic and homogeneous [63]. The synovium is usually thickened without hypervascularity at power Doppler evaluation. Bony irregularities are typically absent (Fig. 5.41).

We must remember that septic arthritis is a great mimic. Polyarticular involvement is very uncommon in septic arthritis [64]. On the contrary, even if the echographic evaluation reveals a monoarticular and homogeneously anechoic effusion, and a synovial thickening without hypervascularity, arthrocentesis is still mandatory if the clinical and laboratory results evoke septic involvement [62].

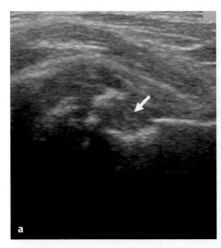
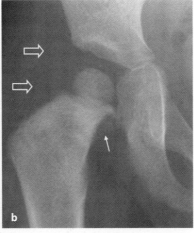

Fig. 5.40 a, b

Septic arthritis of the hip in a limping three-year-old child with mild hip pain. **a** Longitudinal US scan reveals a small effusion with inhomogeneous echogenicity and synovial thickening. Metaphyseal bone erosion is present (*large white arrow*). **b** X-ray in the same patient confirms the soft-tissue swelling around the involved joint, suggestive of effusion (*empty white arrows*), and bone erosion (*small white arrow*)

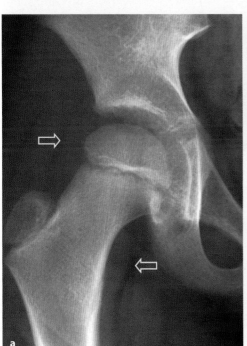
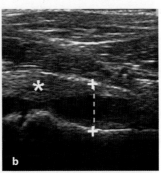
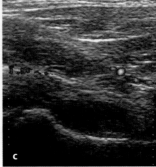

Fig. 5.41 a-c

Transient synovitis in a five-year-old child with similar clinical presentation to that of the patient in Fig. 5.40. **a** Frontal radiograph shows capsular swelling (*empty white arrows*). **b** US detects increased capsule-to-bone distance (*calipers*) related to joint effusion and to synovial thickening (*). **c** Power Doppler US demonstrates absence of intra-synovial increased flow

5.10 Hemophilic arthropathy

Hemophilia is an X-linked recessive bleeding disorder, due to deficiency or absence of blood-clotting factors. It is a disease almost exclusively found in males. Women are asymptomatic carriers and rarely may have acquired hemophilia (immunological origin). Hemorrhagic events may occur from the first years of life and can take place anywhere,

although the musculoskeletal system is the preferred target organ.

US is useful to assess the early stages of hemophilic arthropathy, as it shows synovial proliferation and initial cartilaginous damage [65, 66], not detectable radiologically.

US is also fundamental both for hemorrhage monitoring and evaluation of the response to treatment. The most characteristic clinical manifestation of hemophilia is recurrent hemarthrosis, with secondary chronic synovitis and arthropathy. The knee and elbow are the most commonly involved joints. Recent bleeding appears echogenic, related to the high reflectivity of fresh blood. Later, 48-72 hours after the hemorrhagic event, a progressive decrease in the echogenicity occurs, following blood cell lysis, and the effusion gradually becomes anechoic [16]. Bleeding may occur also in synovial bursae (Fig. 5.42).

Recurrent hemarthrosis can precociously induce villous hyperplasia of the synovium (Fig. 5.43) and, subsequently, a characteristic hemophiliac arthropathy.

Spontaneous bleeding into the muscle is common and may involve any muscle, even in the absence of trauma. The forearm, quadriceps, calf, and iliopsoas are most often involved, the latter having particularly insidious clinical presentation (Fig. 5.44). US evaluation performed within 24-48 hours from symptom onset of the hemorrhage may not be indicative, because recent bleeding usually appears hyperechoic, but sometimes may be isoechoic compared to muscle echogenicity [16]. Later on, the hematoma appears as an anechoic intramuscular area with posterior enhancement.

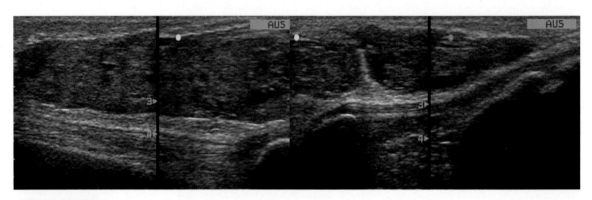

Fig. 5.42

Young male with severe hemophilia. Longitudinal US scan of the anterior aspect of the knee demonstrating enormous distention of the prepatellar bursa by echogenic effusion due to recent bleeding intra-bursal bleeding

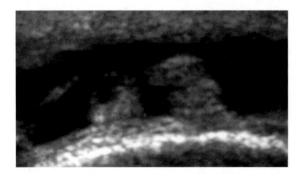

Fig. 5.43

Recurrent hemarthrosis in a patient with hemophilia A. Transverse US scan of the knee depicts the suprapatellar synovial recess which appears distended from abundant anechoic effusion, related to previous hemarthrosis. Synovial villous thickening is also depicted

5.11 Primary and secondary nerve disorders

In several rheumatologic disorders, such as rheumatoid arthritis, polyarteritis nodosa, Wegener's granulomatosis, Churg-Strauss and Sjögren syndrome, one of the clinical landmarks of vasculitis is the appearance of neurological findings [67, 68]. From the pathophysiological point-of-view, the vasculitis-related neuropathy affects large nerve trunks, producing a multifocal degeneration of fibers as a result of necrotizing angiopathy of small nerve arteries, the so called "multiple mononeuropathy" [69]. In these patients, the neuropathy does not correlate with disease parameters (disease activity, rheumatoid factor and functional and radiological scores), and there is sequential involvement of individual nerves both temporally and anatomically [70]. Nerve conduction velocities are

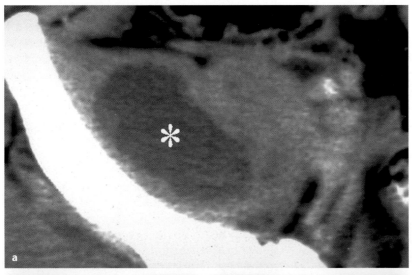

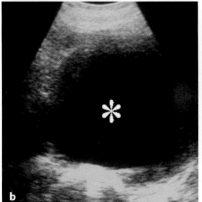
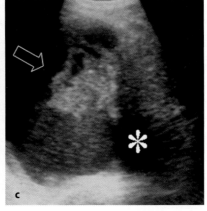

Fig. 5.44 a-c

Patient with severe hemophilia.
a Transverse non-contrast computed tomography (CT) scan detected an old iliopsoas hemorrhage, evident as an intramuscular area of decreased density (*).
b Transverse sonogram in the same patient depicts the echofree appearance of the muscle hemorrhage (*). **c** Echographic reexamination just after sudden recurrence of pain shows the presence of recent bleeding (*empty white arrow*), which appears echogenic and easy to discriminate from the mostly reabsorbed previous hemorrhage (*)

usually not markedly reduced from normal, provided that the compound nerve or muscle action potential is not severely reduced in amplitude [71]. Although multiple mononeuropathy is the most common manifestation, nerve entrapment syndromes may also occur at sites where nerves pass in close proximity to either a synovial joint (i.e. cubital tunnel, tarsal tunnel, Guyon tunnel) or one or more synovial-sheathed tendons (i.e. flexor tendons at the carpal tunnel, flexor hallucis longus at the tarsal tunnel) or para-articular bursae (i.e. iliopsoas bursa at the hip). The clinical evaluation of nerves is often made difficult in these patients by symptoms resulting from pain in the joints and limitations of movement, US imaging can contribute in distinguishing entrapment neuropathies related to derangement of joints and tendon abnormalities (joint effusion, synovial pannus, tophi)

from non-entrapment neuropathy. This is based on the fact that multiple mononeuropathy does not lead to an altered morphology of the affected nerve, whereas entrapment neuropathies do.

Among the individual sites of nerve entrapment, the carpal tunnel is the most commonly involved in patients with rheumatologic disorders. A median nerve area of ≥ 9 mm^2 or ≥ 10 mm^2 calculated at the point of maximum nerve swelling - being just proximal to the edge of the retinaculum or at the scaphoid-pisiform level - has been reported as the best criterion for the diagnosis of carpal tunnel syndrome [72-75]. US also has value in follow-up after surgical release of the retinaculum. After decompression, the appearance of the median nerve may improve even before any definite sign of functional recovery at electrophysiological examination [76].

In rheumatoid arthritis, median nerve compression most often results from amyloid deposits, ganglion cysts or, more commonly, from hypertrophied tenosynovitis of the flexor digitorum tendons (Fig. 5.45). In general, synovial sheath effusion facilitates visualization and differentiation of the individual flexor tendons within the carpal tunnel [77]; dynamic scanning on transverse planes during repetitive flexion and extension movements of the fingers may aid in the differentiation between tendons and echogenic synovium and may reveal restricted passive motion of the compressed nerve beneath the retinaculum. In cases of mild tendon effusion, US scanning should be extended to levels more proximal and distal relative to the carpal tunnel because most synovial fluid may accumulate outside the tunnel.

More rarely, deep synovitis from the radiocarpal and midcarpal joints may lead to anterior displacement of the flexor tendons and compression of the median nerve against the retinaculum. Anomalous bone (lunate) projecting inside the deep portion of the tunnel (often associated with flexor tenosynovitis), can be recognized as the cause of nerve compression as well. This may be secondary to dorsal intercalated instability of the wrist (DISI) following arthritic derangement of the carpal joints and intrinsic carpal ligaments (Fig. 5.46). In these cases, US shows the nerve compressed against the retinaculum by a rounded bony structure bulging from the floor of the carpal tunnel reflecting the displaced lunate. In patients with rheumatoid arthritis and carpal tunnel syndrome, US can help to guide steroid injection within the flexor tendon sheath [78].

At the medial elbow, the ulnar nerve passes in the condylar groove - an osteofibrous tunnel between the olecranon and the medial epicondyle covered by the Osborne retinaculum - and then in the cubital tunnel - a narrow passageway below the aponeurotic arcade between the ulnar and the humeral heads of the flexor carpi ulnaris [77]. Nerve cross-sectional area > 7.5 mm² at the epitrochlear level is considered the threshold value for cubital tunnel syndrome [79]. More recently, a European study based on the normal population revealed that the mean cross-sectional area of this nerve is 7.9 mm² [80]. In patients with overt synovitis of the elbow joint, the nerve may be compressed at the condylar groove or, more often, at the edge of the aponeurosis of the flexor carpi ulnaris by synovial tissue arising from the floor of the tunnel (Fig. 5.47).

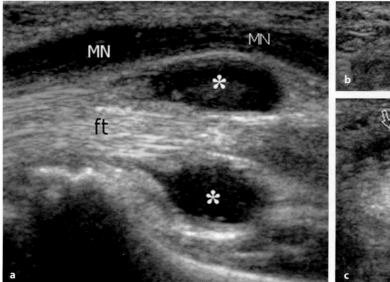
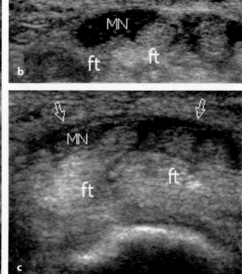

Fig. 5.45 a-c

Carpal tunnel syndrome in tenosynovitis of the flexor tendons. **a** Long-axis US image of the median nerve at the distal radius demonstrates fluid (*) surrounding the flexor tendons (*ft*), resulting in palmar displacement and compression of the median nerve (*MN*) at the entrance of the tunnel. (**b**,**c**) Correlative short-axis US images of the median nerve obtained (**b**) at the distal radius and (**c**) at the proximal tunnel level (scaphoid-pisiform level) show an abnormally enlarged nerve (*MN*) with loss of the fascicular echotexture which becomes flattened behind the flexor retinaculum (*arrows*). Note the convex profile of the retinaculum

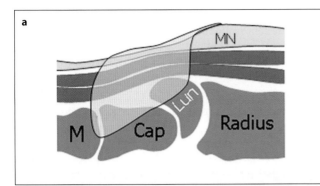
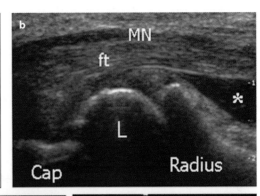
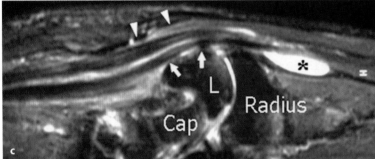
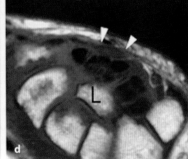

Fig. 5.46 a-d

Carpal tunnel syndrome in long-standing rheumatoid arthritis and dorsal intercalated instability of the wrist (DISI). **a** Schematic drawing over the long axis of the wrist illustrates the mechanism of nerve compression. **b** Longitudinal US image over the proximal carpal tunnel shows the median nerve (*MN*) and the flexor tendons (*ft*) compressed by the prominent lunate (*L*). Within the carpal tunnel, the lunate assumes a crescentic profile (*arrowheads*) due to the volar rotation of its convex articular surface. **c, d** Correlative (**c**) longitudinal fat-suppressed T2-weighted and (**d**) transverse T1-weighted MR images reveal the abnormal position of the lunate (*arrows*) and the median nerve (*arrowheads*) compression against the transverse carpal ligament. *Cap* = capitate; * = effusion

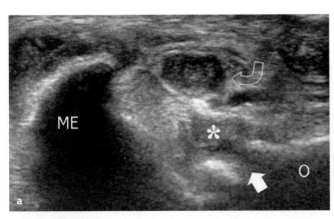
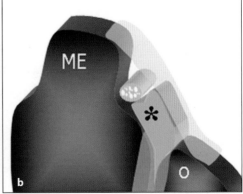

Fig. 5.47 a, b

Cubital tunnel syndrome. **a** Short-axis US image of the cubital tunnel demonstrates the ulnar nerve (*curved arrow*) which appears increasingly swollen and hypoechoic with absent fascicular pattern. Note the irregular appearance of the bony outlines of the medial epicondyle (*ME*) and the olecranon process (*O*) and the elevated floor of the tunnel due to bulging of synovial pannus (*) from the trochlea-ulna joint (*white arrow*). **b** Schematic drawing over the short-axis of the cubital tunnel illustrates the mechanism of nerve compression

Ulnar neuropathy may also result from chronic synovitis, such as in hemophilic arthropathy. In late stage rheumatoid arthritis, some degree of elbow instability related to the inflammatory derangement of joint structures and disruption of the medial collateral ligament or following total elbow arthroplasty may contribute to entrapment of the ulnar nerve in this area [81]. At a more distal location, the ulnar nerve may be occasionally compressed by large effusions arising from the distal radioulnar joint and synovitis around the piso-triquetal joint and the hook of the hamate (Fig. 5.48).

In the lower limb, possible sites of nerve compression include the hip area for the femoral nerve, the popliteal fossa for the peroneal nerve and the tarsal tunnel for the tibial nerve. In the anterior hip, the iliopsoas bursa is a large synovial-lined communicating bursa which lies between the posterior aspect of the iliopsoas muscle and tendon and the anterior capsule of the hip joint [82]. The iliopsoas bursa primarily acts as a reservoir in cases of abundant joint effusions to limit the damage to the intra-articular structures related to a high intra-articular pressure (Fig. 5.49 a). When the bursa is filled with synovial pannus, such as in long-standing rheumatoid arthritis, it appears as a para-articular mass with internal hyperechoic solid components and expand to a large size because of the slow progression of the disease process [83]. With severe joint synovitis the bursa can expand toward the pelvis superficial to the iliopsoas muscle or in between the iliac bone and

the iliacus muscle, possibly causing compression of the femoral nerve that courses under the fascia of the iliacus (Fig. 5.49 b, c) [83, 84].

Somewhat similar to the iliopsoas bursa, the abnormal distension of the semimembranosus-gastrocnemius bursa (Baker cyst) in patients with long-standing rheumatoid arthritis has been reported as a cause of peroneal nerve compression at the posterior knee [85]. At the medial ankle, the tibial nerve and its divisional branches (plantar nerves) travel in the tarsal tunnel between the flexor hallucis longus and the flexor digitorum longus tendons covered by the flexor retinaculum [77]. Because the synovial sheath of the flexor hallucis longus tendon often communicates with the ankle joint, an effusion surrounding this tendon more likely reflects the joint disease rather than a tendon abnormality, especially when considerable ankle joint involvement is present. In these cases, the nerve may be stretched and entrapped by the distended sheath in the retromalleolar region. Marked distension of the medial recesses of the subtalar joint by synovial pannus and effusion may also cause extrinsic compression and disturbances of tibial nerve function (Fig. 5.50).

Diabetes mellitus is one of systemic disorders associated with neuropathy. In this disorder, nerves are more vulnerable as they traverse osteofibrous tunnels. In diabetic patients with tarsal tunnel syndrome, the cross-sectional area of the tibial nerve is significantly larger compared with normal subjects and asymptomatic diabetics [86].

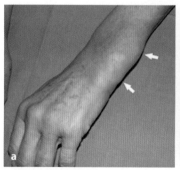 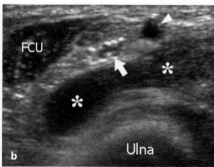 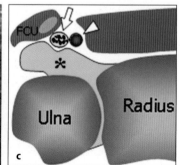

Fig. 5.48 a-c

Ulnar neuropathy secondary to marked synovitis of the distal radioulnar joint and mild symptoms of ulnar neuropathy. **a** Photograph demonstrates considerable soft-tissue swelling (*arrows*) over the dorsoulnar aspect of the patient's wrist. **b** Transverse US image over the ventral aspect of the wrist reveals prominent synovitis (*) leading to displacement of the ulnar nerve (*arrow*) against the flexor carpi ulnaris (*FCU*). **c** Schematic drawing correlation. *Arrowhead* = ulnar artery

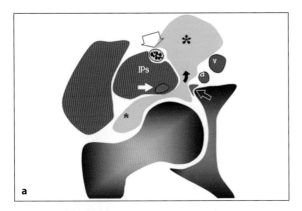
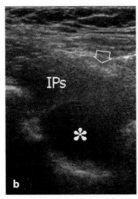
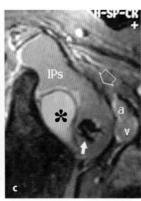

Fig. 5.49 a-c

Femoral neuropathy related to hip joint synovitis. **a** Iliopsoas bursitis. Schematic drawing of a transverse view through the hip illustrates the mechanism of compression of the femoral nerve (*large arrow*) by an effusion located within the iliopsoas synovial bursa (*). The joint cavity communicates with the bursa through a thin pedicle (*curved arrow*). Note the anterior recess filled with fluid, the iliopsoas muscle (IPs) and tendon (white arrow). *Empty arrow* = anterosuperior labrum; *a* = femoral artery; *b* = femoral vein. **b** Transverse US image with (**c**) GRE T2* MR imaging correlation over the anterior inferior iliac spine reveals proximal migration of the synovitis (*) leading to an indirect compression of the femoral nerve (*empty arrow*) which courses under the fascia of the iliacus muscle

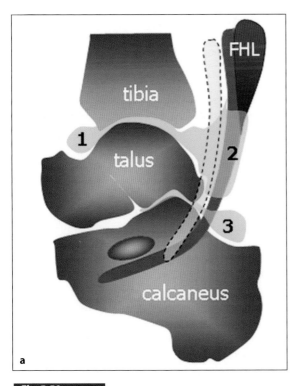
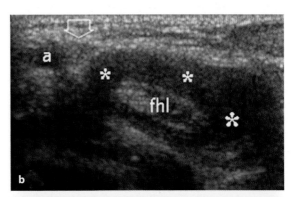
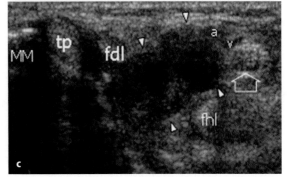

Fig. 5.50 a-c

Tarsal tunnel syndrome. **a** Schematic drawing of a sagittal view through the ankle illustrates the relationships of the tibial nerve (*dashed lines*) with the anterior (1) and posterior (2) recesses of the ankle joint, the posterior recess of the subtalar joint (3) and the flexor hallucis longus (FHL). Note the communication between the posterior recess of the ankle joint and the sheath of the flexor hallucis longus. **b** Tibial neuropathy in a patient with rheumatoid arthritis and remarkable distension of the sheath (*) of the FHL tendon by synovial pannus. The tibial nerve (*arrow*) and the posterior tibial artery (*a*) appear displaced by the synovial process. **c** Tibial neuropathy in a patient with rheumatoid arthritis and marked subtalar joint synovitis. Note the synovial tissue (*arrowheads*) as it projects within the tarsal tunnel between the flexor digitorum longus (FDL) and the FHL tendons leading to a displacement of the tibial nerve (*arrow*) and the posterior tibial artery (*a*) and vein (*v*). *tp* = tibialis posterior; *MM* = medial malleolus

5.12 Sport and rheumatology

The musculoskeletal system of athletes is submitted to continuous stress, both during training and when competing, so that it is exposed to the risk of trauma. A post-traumatic injury occurs when the athletic exercise involves a movement that overcomes the resistance limit of a musculo-tendinous structure, ligament, bone or joint. Exceeding resistance threshold of a specific anatomical structure may be caused both by acute (macrotraumas) pathogenetic mechanisms and chronic (repeated microtraumas). In the first case, the injury is the result of a repeated highly energetic movement carried out by the athlete, that eventually produces functional overload (overuse syndrome). The repetitive performance of an incorrect athletic movement promotes the occurrence of the lesion, especially in inexperienced and poorly trained athletes, or in athletes presenting with pre-existing musculoskeletal conditions which reduce the resistance threshold to mechanical load.

Acute lesions, instead, occur in a precise mechanical moment (falls or direct impacts) that produces immediate and painful lesions that necessitate interruption of the sport activity.

Lesions can therefore be divided into two types:
- Chronic lesions due to repeated functional overload (overuse syndromes).
- Acute lesions caused by macrotraumas (falls or direct impacts).

Functional overload pathology

Functional overload pathologies, or overuse syndromes, correspond to a range of musculoskeletal system conditions caused by a single pathogenetic mechanism represented by a continual microtraumatic event occurring repeatedly on the same anatomical region. Repeated and highly intense athletic movement alters the delicate balance between the necessary working load for training and the capability of biological and mechanical functional recovery. Therefore, the continual repetition of some athletic movements can lead to a specific musculoskeletal condition, characterized by the overlap of several repeated microlesions. The lesions caused by microtraumas can accumulate because they are asymptomatic in early phases and it is only later that they present with pain and sometimes with functional limitation. A microtraumatic event occurs when the load applied to an anatomical structure overcomes its resistance limit. If energy remains the same, the severity of the lesion is inversely proportional to the resistance limit of the structure. Obviously an anatomical structure already damaged by previous microtraumas is more easily exposed to the risk of new lesions. Similarly, systemic metabolic and rheumatic conditions, together with ageing, may weaken some body regions and make them easy targets for micro- or macrotraumas [87]. In such cases, while evaluating a pathologic finding, the sonographer should always consider a differential diagnosis of simple functional overload cause, pre-existing rheumatologic cause or both.

The functional overload may involve a bone segment, a joint or, more frequently, a musculo-tendinous functional unit.

The most frequent pathological findings in sport-related overuse syndromes are represented by **tendon degenerative and inflammatory diseases**, **enthesopathies** and **bursitis**. US is the imaging technique of first choice for the evaluation of an athlete's musculo-tendinous pathology. In tendinopathy the US appearance has a non-specific pattern and cannot be distinguished from analogous tendinopathies. Specific features in athletes include the lesion location, the performed athletic movement and the type of sport activity. The application of power and color Doppler techniques is useful because it adds important "functional" information on tendon perfusion and allows the evaluation of therapy response. The "functional" information is derived from the intensity of signal found.

Insertional tendinopathy of adolescent athletes has more specific characteristics. During growth the weakest anatomical region is found at the cartilage growth plate, where functional overload can causes damage to the growing cartilage (**apophysitis**) rather than tendinopathy. The typical alteration associated with apophysitis is represented by chondritis and consequent alteration of the growing enchondral ossification center, which appears typically fragmented.

A **stress fracture** may occur when athletic movements are performed repeatedly over a long period of time and at increased working loads.

Bone is a biologically active tissue with slow metabolism, and repairs lesions over a longer time than muscles and other tissues with faster metabolism. Even physiological load in sport, when repeated over a long period of time and in the presence of intrinsic (for example, size of a bone segment) and extrinsic (type of shoes, ground, etc.) factors, can be responsible for lesions involving the musculoskeletal system and particularly bone. When an excessive load is applied to a bone segment and the requested adaptation overcomes normal physiology resorption activity may outweigh the formation of new bone until a fracture occurs. A stress fracture is diagnosed when a fracture line is detected on a plain radiograph. Stress fractures alone represent 10% of all sport injuries. Considering this high incidence, the role of radiology is very important in detecting stress fractures because there are several conditions to be considered as differential diagnosis (tendinopathies, reactive periostitis, muscular lesions,

tumors). The distribution of lesions changes according to the type of activity and the specific athletic movement. The tarsal scaphoid is often injured in track and field specialties that involve hurdles and jumping; metatarsal and pelvic bones in running, mainly long distance; tibia and fibula in sprints, middle distance and hurdling.

Osteo-cartilagineous lesions or associated canalicular syndromes may be caused by excessive and repeated articular impact; similarly repeated friction may involve a nearby nervous structure.

Particularly in early phases, a conventional radiograph may show no fracture line; in this case it is necessary to perform further investigations such as scintigraphy, CT and particularly MR imaging. US has very limited usefulness because it can only rarely confirm fracture with the typical irregular cortical focus surrounded by a hypoechoic paraosteal edema and sometimes, a defined periosteal reaction thickening (Fig. 5.51).

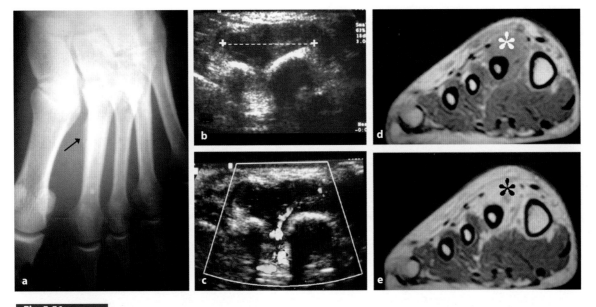

Fig. 5.51 a-e

Stress fracture of the diaphisis of 2nd metatarsal bone. **a** The plain film shows the periostal reaction (*arrow*) at the site of fracture. The fracture line cannot be seen. **b** Standard US examination shows a hypoechoic halo (*calipers*) that wraps the 2nd and part of the 3rd metatarsal bone. This is related to soft tissue edema. **c** The color Doppler scan shows a color spot inside the paraosteal edema. The MR scan T1 W, pre- and post-gadolinium) shows the metatarsal periostosis at the site of fracture and the paraosteal edema (*). It appears hypointense before gadolinium (**d**) and hyperintense after gadolinium (**e**) (courtesy of Dott. Antonio Barile)

Pathologic conditions

Lower limb

In runners, overuse syndromes exclusively affect the lower limb. Overload lesions consist almost exclusively of insertional tendinopathies and US is the investigation of choice. The following tendon insertions may develop overuse syndromes: the *rectus femoris muscle* insertion on the antero-inferior iliac crest (Fig. 5.52), the *adductor muscles* (responsible for pubalgia) and the *flexor muscles* of the knee (the socalled *hamstring* muscles). All of these cases have a US pattern consisting of typical insertional tendinopathy, in which the insertional tract appears thickened, inhomogeneous and hypoechoic and may show intratendinous pre-insertional calcification at a late stage [88]. MR imaging is necessary in therapy-resistant cases, to detect possible inflammatory involve-

ment of the bone at the tendon insertion (*stress response*) [89].

A very common tendinopathy in competitive athletes as well as amateurs, is *Achilles tendinopathy* [90]. There can be several conditions that involve the Achilles tendon, such as tendinitis, tendinosis, mixed forms (peritendinitis occurring on tendinosis), tendon ruptures and enthesopathies, but they can vary from patient to patient, depending on the evolutional phase of the pathology [91]. US is able to correctly identify tendon structure alteration and possible associated deep infracalcaneal bursitis and/or a superficial retrocalcaneal bursitis [92]. The power Doppler technique complements the standard US examination and can detect the degree of inflammatory hyperemia (and its change at follow-up), together with identyfing the peritendinitis and differentiate it from the mixed form of peritendinitis occurring on tendi-

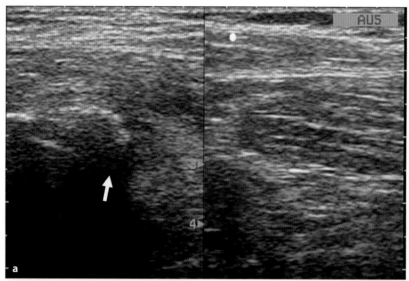

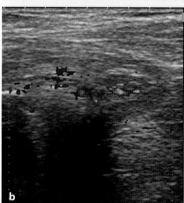

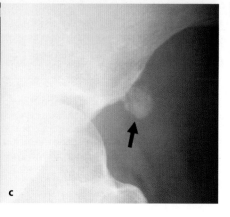

Fig. 5.52 a-c

Insertional tendinopathy of rectus femoris on the antero-inferior iliac crest. **a** The longitudinal US scan shows complete disarray of the tendon echotexture with rough calcification (*arrow*). **b** The power Doppler scan, complementing the information obtained with grayscale US shows some vascular spots, related to inflammatory hyperemia. **c** The plain film shows the insertional calcific metaplasia of the tendon (*arrow*) on the antero-inferior iliac crest

nosis (Fig.5.53) [93-95]. In addition, the US diagnosis of Achilles overuse syndrome is of great importance, because it represents a severe risk factor for the spontaneous rupture of the tendon itself. Factors predicting rupture are the presence of focal hypoechoic zones and sagittal tendon thickness greater than 10 mm.

Such a US pattern may suggest that the rheumatologist includes metabolic causes of tendinosis in the differential diagnosis, such as gout and hypercholesterolemia. Both conditions cause thickening of the Achilles tendon due to the accumulation of deposits of uric acid and cholesterol, respectively (tendon xanthomatosis).

With the advent of US the role of conventional radiology for the study of achillodynia and thallodynia has diminished and has been exclusively directed to the study of bone for the detection of postero-superior calcaneal tuberosity hypertrophies (Haglund disease). This anatomical variant promotes the onset of insertional Achilles tendinopathy, which is often associated with bursitis and edema of the calcaneal spongy bone at the insertion site (Fig.4.40).

It should be kept in mind that an Achilles enthesopathy may be the sign of a systemic enthesoarthritis, such as psoriatic arthritis and Reiter disease, whose onset may be the consequence of mechanical impact; this hypothesis should be particularly considered in case of bilateral achillodynia and of past arthralgia and enthesalgia, even if just transitory and in other sites (Fig. 5.54).

In these cases, the role of ultrasound is to detect the presence of an enthesitis in early phases, showing reduced echoes and a clear increase of the thickness at the insertional tract compared to the mid-distal tract. The comparison of the two sides usually does not add information since the condition may be symmetrical and bilateral [96]. The plain radiograph can be instead very useful to detect calcaneal spurs in more advanced phases.

Ilio-tibial band inflammation, also known as "marathon runner's knee", is a syndrome represented by the friction of these structures on the lateral femoral epicondyle, caused by repeated flexion/extension of the knee during running. This syndrome is characterized by pain along the lateral aspect of the knee, so that a condition affecting the lateral meniscus should be considered in the differential diagnosis. The inflammation may first involve only the ilio-tibial band and afterwards spread around the nearby soft tissues and the synovial bursae.

The ilio-tibial band appears at ultrasound as a hyperechoic lamellar structure adjacent to the lat-

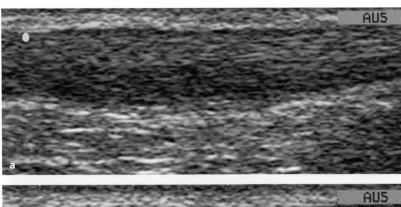

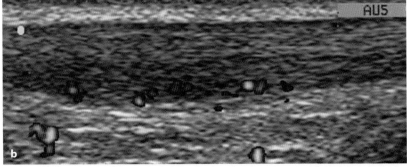

Fig. 5.53 a, b

Fusiform thickening of the Achilles tendon with disarray of the fibrillar echotexture typical of tendinosis (**a**). The power Doppler scan (**b**) shows several color spots depending on the peritendinous inflammatory hyperemia

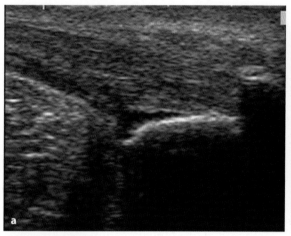
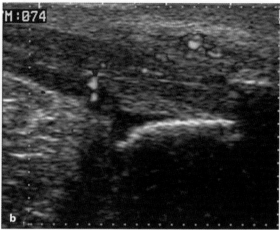

Fig. 5.54 a, b

Enthesopathy of the Achilles tendon. **a** The longitudinal scan shows inhomogeneous echotexture and thickening of the pre-insertional portion of the tendon, on a degenerative basis, with a rough calcaneal spur. Chronic inflammation of the superficial retrocalcaneal bursa with soft tissue thickening is also shown. **b** The color Doppler scan confirms inflammation of the retrocalcaneal bursa and shows many vascular spots in the tendon

eral femoral condyle but, when it is involved in a inflammatory process, it appears thickened and hypoechoic, and often associated with a synovial reaction found between the band and the femoral condyle [97].

In jumpers, overload related musculo-tendinous injuries mainly affect the extensor tendons of the knee, producing the so-called *jumper's knee*. The clinical findings often consist of well localised pain, usually at the lower extremity of the patella, exacerbated by physical activity. The most common site of disease is in fact the proximal insertion of the patellar tendon (about 65% of cases), followed by the superior patellar extremity (25%) and the tibial tuberosity (10%). An accurate history together with clinical data, are often sufficient to derive a diagnosis. The role of diagnostic imaging is still of great importance to exclude the presence of other pathologic conditions presenting with anterior knee pain, often coexisting in these patients, such as bursitis, meniscal pathologies, chondromalacia or pathologies, chondromalacia or Hoffa's fat pad pathology. US is the technique of choice to define the degree of the tendon lesion [98]. Two different conditions can be detected by US: an insertional tendinopathy or a tendinosis, either singularly or co-existant.

Insertional tendinopathy is responsible for pain and it is also the most frequent (about 92% of cases). At US the tendon is inhomogeneous and

hypoechoic at its insertional tract, where it appears thickened and widened with a fan-like shape (Fig. 1.13). Hypoechoic foci can be observed at the osteo-tendinous junction, reported to be focal microtears (Fig. 5.56).

In tendinosis, a condition that promotes tendon rupture, the patellar tendon is extensively tickened and inhomogeneously hypoechoic, sometimes showing pre-insertional intratendinous calcification [99].

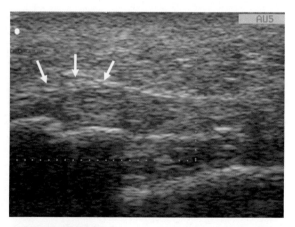

Fig. 5.55

Longitudinal scan of the sole of the foot showing inflammatory thickening (*arrows*) of the plantar fascia at its calcaneal insertion

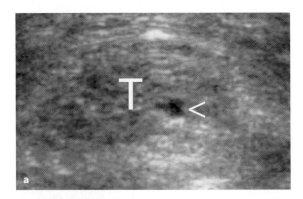
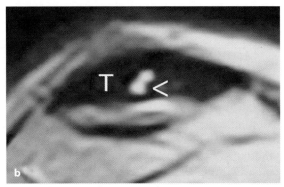

Fig. 5.56 a, b

a This longitudinal scan of the proximal third of the patellar tendon (*T*) shows diffuse disarray of the fibrillar echotexture with a small, well-defined, hypoechoic area (*arrowheads*), related to a partial tear. **b** The MR scan of the same patient (T2 W turbo spin echo (TSE)) confirms the diagnosis (hyperintense area, *arrowhead*)

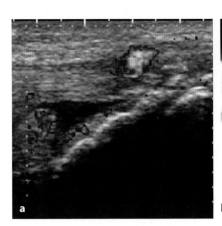
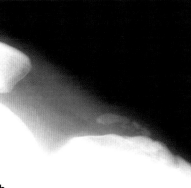

Fig. 5.57 a, b

Osgood-Schlatter's disease. **a** Ultrasound allows assessment of the morphostructural alterations of the distal insertion of patellar tendon, the inflammatory distension of the deep pretibial bursa and the unevenness of anterior tibial apophysis. Power Doppler scan shows a mild hyperemia on the bursal wall and at the tendon insertion. **b** Plain film of the same patient

In the enthesis of pediatric patients, the apophyseal cartilage growth plate is a less resistant site in the muscle-tendon-bone functional/ anatomical unit. The mechanical overload occurring in athletes during growth is concentrated almost exclusively on the growth plate, sparing other anatomical sites. For this reason, tendon and ligament injuries are extremely rare in children and adolescents, while overuse syndromes are more frequent and show up with apophysitis. At the knee this may involve the anterior tibial tuberosity (Osgood-Schlatter's disease) or the inferior patellar extremity (Sinding-Larsen-Johansson's syndrome). Both syndromes are characterized by chondritis at the tendon insertion close to the apophyseal ossification center; the growing cartilage shows increased thickness and strong chondro-tendinous junction hyperemia is observed at power Doppler. An adjacent bursitis can be associated. The inflammatory hyperemia together with incorrect repeated movements may cause altered enchondral ossification, and the calcified center may appear bulky and fragmented (Fig. 5.57).

Upper limb

The *painful shoulder syndrome* in sport is usually a condition secondary to chronic microtrauma acting on the rotator cuff and on the long head of biceps. This condition affects mainly competitive athletes in overhead disciplines, in which the repeated athletic task carried out by the arm has to overcome the acromion-clavicular plane (volleyball, handball, throwing, water polo, swimming, tennis, gymnastics, weightlifting) [100].

Repeated and powerful athletic task, consistent with throwing specialties, produces continual traction overload on the rotator cuff tendons, particularly supraspinatus. The final pathological outcome consists of functional loss of supraspinatus that no longer acts to actively stabilize the shoulder and keep the humeral head in position. Consequently, the humeral head tends to go up with friction and impact against the acromial vault. The resulting coraco-acromial impingement syndrome causes a further worsening of the rotator cuff tendinopathy. This pathological condition evolves from a simple insertional tendinopathy of the supraspinatus to a tendinosis followed by rupture. The long head of biceps (tenosynovitis - tendinosis) and the subdeltoid bursa (acute bursitis - chronic bursitis) can also be involved [101]. In some sports, such as water polo, which involve maximum external rotation and abduction movements, other types of impingements, such as the postero-superior impingement; and coraco-humeral impingement (also know as antero-internal impingement) can occur [102].

Another pathological condition caused by shoulder overuse is the *long head of biceps tendon or dislocation* (Fig. 4.49). This condition is often associated with other lesions involving adjacent structures, such as a complete or partial rupture of the subscapular tendon or, more rarely, an isolated rupture of the coracohumeral ligament [103].

In shoulder pain the diagnostic path is chosen mainly depends according to the patient's age and clinical presentation. Initial investigations include conventional radiology and US looking for calcium deposits in peri-articular soft tissues, and the site and the severity of the main injury affecting tendons and/or bursa respectively (Fig.5.58). A stable, non-surgical, painful shoulder, therefore, can be monitored with conservative therapy by means of US, complemented by power Doppler [104].

In case of a young competitive athlete presenting with unstable painful shoulder, the gold standard examination is arthroMRI, which is the only investigation able to point out a possible injury to bones, glenoid labrum, intracapsular tendons and ligaments.

A well-known example of tendinopathy affecting the upper limb is "tennis elbow", consisting of edema and swelling of the common epicondylar insertion of the extensor-supinator muscles and particularly of the extensor carpi radialis brevis. The epitrochleitis, also known as "golfer's elbow", is the most common cause of pain reported at the medial aspect of the elbow with involvement of the common epitrochlear insertion of the flexor/pronator muscles. A correct diagnosis of epitrochleitis is usually made with an accurate history together with an attentive clinical examination. Diagnostic imaging, including conventional radiograms, US and MRI, can be used as a complement to the clinical findings or in therapy-resistant cases. Plain film may show insertional calcifications and bone erosions.

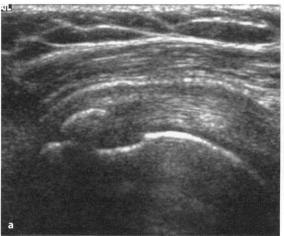
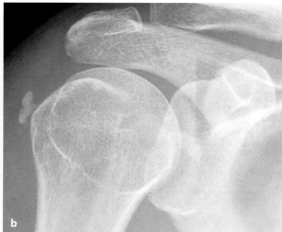

Fig. 5.58 a, b

Rough calcification of the supraspinatus tendon at its insertion. **a** US and (**b**) plain film

US is able to detect insertional tendon thickening and corresponding degenerative alteration, appearing as hypoechoic spots often associated with an irregular appearance of the cortical bone and with intratendinous micro and macrocalcifications [105]. The use of Doppler techniques can add further information regarding the inflammatory hyperemia (Fig.5.59).

It is important to keep in mind that when facing therapy-resistant cases (4-10% of all cases), the physician should verify that the epicondylar pain is not due to a ligament injury in an unstable elbow; in such cases an MR examination should be performed. US is also able to confirm the hypothesis of bursal inflammation and identify contents (plain fluid in reactive and post-traumatic collections, corpuscular fluid in bacterial collections, complicated by synechiae and synovial hyperplasia in rheumatic conditions). Power Doppler analysis of the synovial proliferation allows further information on the presence and amplitude of inflammatory hypertermia.

In athletes performing repeated throwing insertional wrist tendinopathy is observed in some cases, particularly affecting the *flexor carpi ulnaris*, an anchor tendon inserting onto the pisiform. US may show focal thickening of the tendon at its insertion on the pisiform and disrray of the typical fibrillar pattern [107].

De Quervain's disease is a tenosynovitis of the 1st compartment of extensors, or rather of the abductor longus and extensor pollicis brevis tendons, as they run along the radial styloid. The pathogenesis relates to overuse of the thumb or wrist, caused by continual friction against the corresponding retinaculum. This often follows repeated and abrupt movements of abduction of the thumb and of ulnar deviation of the wrist (such as skiing and other sports involving the use of poles) [108]. The US pattern of De Quervain's disease is strictly related to its clinical stage. The early US finding consists of non-specific exudative tenosynovitis, mildly hyperemic on power Doppler analysis. In advanced, chronic stages, the main pattern is that of tendinosis, while the inflammatory component appears hypertrophic rather than exudative and, typically, the retinaculum gets thicker thereby worsening the impingement with tunderlying tendons (chronic stenosing tenosynovitis) (Fig.5.60).

About 4-6 cm proximal to the radial styloid, the 1st compartment extensor tendons intersect the 2nd compartment tendons (extensor carpi radialis brevis and longus), forming a critical anatomical area for the possible onset of *intersection syndrome*. This syndrome consists of a tenosynovitis affecting patients that carry out a continual flexion and extension of the wrist, such as weightlifters or rowers, and it is clinically characterized by local pain and swelling. The US pattern is characterized by

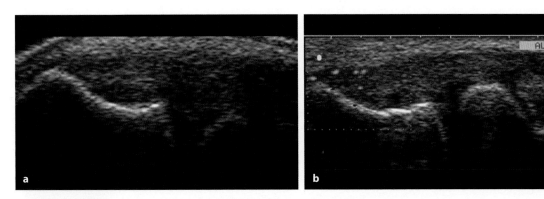

Fig. 5.59 a, b

Lateral epicondylitis (tennis elbow). **a** The common extensor tendon appears thickened and inhomogeneous, on a degenerative basis. **b** Power Doppler shows vascular spots at the common extensor tendon insertion

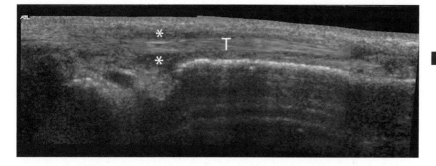

Fig. 5.60

The longitudinal extended field of view (*EFOV*) US scan obtained at the wrist shows a tenosynovitis of the first compartment of the extensors. The sheath (*) is thickened while the tendon structures are intact (*T*)

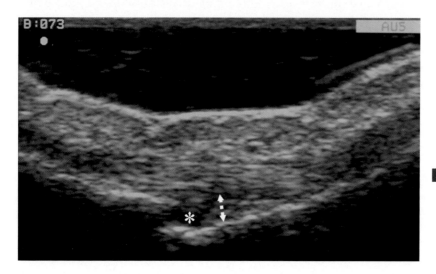

Fig. 5.61

The longitudinal US scan of flexor tendons obtained at the finger shows separation of the tendon from the underlying bone (*arrows*), following a rupture of a pulley. Note the fluid (*)

typical tenosynovial exudative inflammation of the corresponding tendons.

Tenosynovitis of the wrist *flexor tendons* may result in *carpal tunnel syndrome*. Even if this is one of the less common causes of carpal tunnel syndrome related to sports, it is still important to evaluate. *Trigger finger (or Notta-Nelaton's disease)* is a very common disorder consisting of painful clicking that occurs when trying to flex or extend a finger. The pathology of trigger finger is related to a chronic stenosing tenosynovitis affecting the flexor digitorum tendons at the first flexor pulley level. In these cases, a dynamic US examination is very useful to highlight the pseudo-nodular thickening of the tendon sheath.

In rock-climbing, the hand and wrist can be affected by several overuse injuries, the detection of which is essential to correct therapy and to prevent possible severe functional impairment.

The most common overuse syndrome is the flexor tenosynovitis, in which the patient cannot actively flex his/her finger (passive flexion is usually preserved). US is able to demonstrate tendon sheath involvement with assessment of the condition of the tendons and pulleys (whether or not ruptures and/or avulsions have occurred) allows either conservative or surgical therapy to be correctly chosen (Fig. 5.61).

Acute traumatic pathology

Traumatic pathology in sport is an important and extremely interesting subject for the rheumatologist. Athletes are always running the risk of trauma, often occurring by accident, but sometimes due to poor training or to a lack of correct pre-exercise warm-up. Therefore, non-competitive athletes are also exposed to the risk of musculo-skeletal traumas and it is important that rheumatologists, while deriving a diagnosis, keep in mind "sport trauma".

When assessing an acute injury, plain films and US are the imaging techniques of first choice, the latter allows an accurate evaluation of soft tissues, tendons, muscles and ligaments.

Trauma can be classified as follows:
- direct trauma (contusions and impacts);
- indirect trauma (caused by incorrect distribution of mechanical forces: falls, sprains, abrupt or incorrect movements).

Sport-related trauma can produce:
- muscular injuries;
- tendinous injuries;
- ligamentous injuries;
- joint dislocation;
- bone fractures.

We should keep in mind that all the listed conditions may coexist. In addition, an acute injury can occur within a pre-existing chronic condition.

Acute traumatic pathologies and overuse syndromes should not then be considered different clinical conditions, but two entities that can coexist in the same clinical situation.

Muscular lesions

Acute muscular injuries are the most common lesions occurring in sport-related trauma, with an incidence varying from 10% to 30% of all sport traumas. They are often observed in sports involving running, jumping, abrupt changes of direction and physical contact with other athletes.

Adequate athletic training and pre-exercise warm-up are very important to prevent the occurrence of muscular injuries. There are several factors affecting the occurrence of a trauma, such as a high ratio between muscular belly volume and tendon length, past injury and degenerative disease. Extrinsic factors such as the sport ground hardness, the type of shoes, the temperature and many others should be considered.

A muscular injury can be produced in two ways:
- contusion or direct trauma: occurs when an object strongly hits the muscle (the more contracted the muscle at the impact, the more severe the lesion);
- sprain or indirect trauma: is more common and depends on an abnormal distribution of the mechanical forces on the muscular fibers.

The difference between contusion-derived and sprain-derived muscular ruptures is not limited to the pathogenetic mechanism, but is also based on the clinical findings and on the evolution (more favorable in sprain-derived ruptures).

Muscle ruptures, in both cases, can be classified into three degrees of severity of the injury that has occurred, directly proportional to the clinical presentation [109].

A **strain rupture** occurs when a sudden pull of the muscular fibers, over their resistance limit, causes tears in the critical weak areas. The most commonly exposed muscles are pennate bi-articular muscles and those muscles with a high white fiber density, whose critical areas consist of the central myo-aponeurotic junction, the myofascial junction, the myotendinous junction and the osteo-muscular junction.

In a **1st degree** strain injury only a few fibers are torn within one or some fascicles. Blood extravasation may not be observed (*distention*) or it may be very minor (*minor distraction*).

A **2nd degree** strain injury (Fig. 5.62) corresponds to laceration of one or more fascicles, involving less than three quarters of the anatomical section of the muscle at the injured level. As a rule, between the lesional edges a hematoma is found, which appears isoechoic during the first 24 hours and becomes hypo-anechoic 24-48 hours after the traumatic event. Follow-up examinations show a hyperechoic wall, growing thicker and thicker until it fills the cavity.

A **3rd degree** strain injury corresponds to a lesion involving more than three quarters of the anatomical section of the muscle at the injured level (*severe strain*), including complete rupture with retraction of the stumps (Fig. 5.63). Blood collection is usually considerable and fills the rupture cavity. The covering fascia may be preserved, although in most cases the hematoma extends by passing through a laceration.

Muscle contusions may present with different US patterns, usually according to the degree of the injury. A 2nd and 3rd degree contusion rupture correspond to severe muscular injury showing irregular muscular fiber tears, inhomogeneously thickened by blood infarction, with a large hematoma occupying the intervening space. At the site of impact increased thickness of the skin and of the subcutaneous tissue can be observed. The muscular fascia (usually seen as a hyperechoic line) shows an irregular pattern. In acute

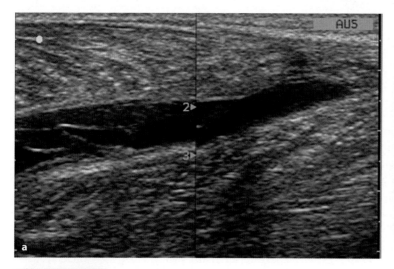
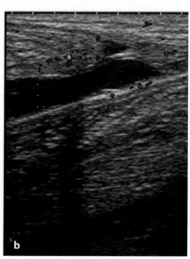

Fig. 5.62 a, b

a Subacute grade II tear of the medial gastrocnemius at the tenomuscular junction. Note the hematoma in the tear between gastrocnemius and soleus. **b** Power Doppler analysis shows the reactive hyperemia in the bellies

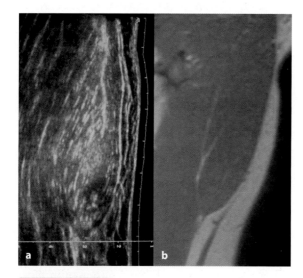

Fig. 5.63 a, b

Result of a grade III tear of the abductor longus muscle. **a** The EFV US scan shows the cranial retraction of the fibres. **b** MR scan of the same patient (SE T1W)

phases, the high echoes from the hematoma may limit assessment of the lesion, by underestimating its actual dimensions. 48-72 hours after the trauma, the collection becomes diffusely anechoic, allowing correct measurement of the lesion. When evaluating the healing at follow-up, US will show progressive resorption of the blood collection and hyperechoic tissue filling the lesion from the periphery to the center.

US is extremely important to define the type of muscle injury and the site and degree of the lesion, so that a correct therapeutic plan and an accurate prognostic evaluation can be made. US also has a fundamental role in follow-up, when assessing healing.

When muscle injuries are not correctly treated they can result in an unfavorable outcome with severe sequelae. US can detect fibrous scars (Fig. 4.57), sero-hemorragic cysts and myositis ossificans. Scar tissue has a hypoechoic appearance and an acoustic shadow can be seen behind the areas affected by myositis ossificans, identifiable with ultrasound at earlier stages than with conventional radiology (Fig. 4.55).

Less commonly, as a result of sport-related trauma (for example a violent blow hitting the thigh or the leg), an **acute compartmental syndrome** consisting of compression of vascular and nervous structures by edema and hematoma can develop. US assessment of the adjacent vascularity complemented with color Doppler techniques, is fundamental for the differential diagnosis. Compartmental syndrome is more frequently derived from prolonged strain (Delayed-Onset Muscle Soreness (DOMS)), as seen in long distance runners or after repeated violent impacts on a body region. In these cases, the volume of muscle involved is increased by edema, with a inhomogeneous increase in basal echogenicity wich can hide the regular myofibrillar echoes.

Tendon and ligament tears

Rupture of a tendon can be the result of direct penetrating trauma or indirect trauma caused by excessive loading during physical activity. In athletes, injury of a tendon is usually related to a pre-existing degenerative condition of the tendon itself.

A typical example of this kind of injury is the rupture of the distal segment of the biceps tendon that, when the rupture is complete, can be retracted proximally to the elbow [110].

Likewise, the quadriceps and patellar tendons can be damaged by violent distraction of the extensor system of the knee, which can result in rupture at their insertion. Most tears occur at the myotendinous junction, while a small amount of them occur in the parenchyma. For instance, the Achilles tendon can be torn at the myotendinous junction, in the parenchyma, or at the enthesis, though the common site of rupture is 4 to 6 cm from its insertion onto the calcaneum. This is an area of relative weakness because of the poor vascularization of the region (critical area) (Fig 5.64) [111]. A critical area is also present on the pre-insertional segment of supraspinatus.

When evaluating a tendon lesion plain film findings are usually poor, non-specific or limited to small bony detachments. Radiological confirmation of a tendon tear must be performed by the application of more specific and sensitive imaging techniques, such as US and MR [112]. The most common site of tendon rupture is the insertion onto the bone and, in adults, this can result in small bony avulsion whilst in children and teenagers these lesions may result in partial or complete detachment of the corresponding growing cartilage. In this last case, ultrasound must be complemented with a plain film or with a CT or MR scan if doubt persists.

Ligaments are often involved in sport traumas and must be carefully assessed because their rupture can often lead to instability of the involved joint. In acute conditions, clinical examination is difficult to perform because of the effusion, pain and muscular contraction: these patients can be easily examined with US. If the ligament is partially torn, the involved segment appears hypoechoic and thickened (Fig. 5.65).

In complete ruptures, the ligament appears discontinuous and its stumps are separated by hematoma appearing anechoic or hypoechoic according to the time passed since the traumatic event (Fig. 4.53).

It is important to keep in mind that US can assess superficial ligaments but not deep ones; moreover, it cannot detect any other lesions occurring at the same time, such as meniscal tears, osteochondral lesions, hidden fractures or bone edema. These lesions must be assessed with a CT or a MR scan.

A particularly important example of ligament tear for the rheumatologist is that involving is the *ulnar collateral ligament* (UCL). Moreover, rheumatoid arthritis may cause partial or complete tears of the UCL. Clinical findings and diagnostic imaging are extremely important to reach a final diagnosis. A reported history of violent trauma with the

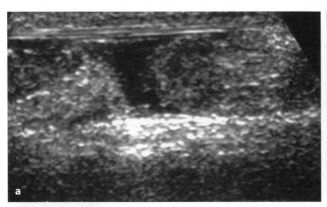 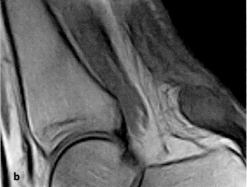

Fig. 5.64 a, b

Subcutaneous complete rupture of a degenerative Achilles tendon. **a** The US scan shows a complete tear. Note the effusion between the stumps. **b** The MR scan confirms the diagnosis (SE T1W)

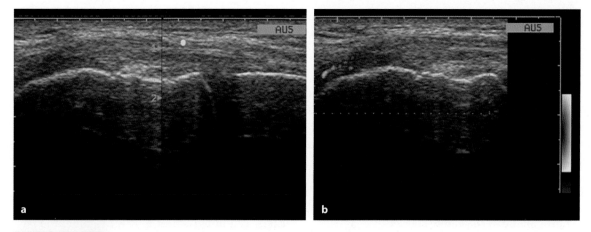

Fig. 5.65 a, b

Grade II tear of the medial collateral ligament of the knee (long axis view). **a** The ligament appears continuous but thickened and inhomogeneous. **b** Power Doppler analysis shows reactive hyperemia at the deep fibers of the femoral insertion

thumb being extremely abducted and hyperextended is very important when considering a differential diagnosis. Nowadays, MRI and US are the most accurate investigative techniques for the assessment of the integrity of the ulnar collateral ligament. US may only detect the superficial hematoma and edema [113]. Stenner's lesion refers to a complete tear of the UCL associated with retraction of the proximal end, appearing dislocated over the tendon aponeurosis insertion of the abductor pollicis. Avulsions may also occur, more commonly at the distal insertion (medial aspect of the base of the proximal phalanx) rather than proximal (1st metacarpal head).

References

1. Grassi W, Salaffi F, Filippucci E (2005) Ultrasound in rheumatology. Best Pract Res Clin Rheumatol 19:467-485
2. Grassi W, Filippucci E, Busilacchi P (2004) Musculoskeletal ultrasound. Best Pract Res Clin Rheumatol 18:813-826
3. Kane D, Balint PV, Sturrock R, Grassi W (2004) Musculoskeletal ultrasound-a state of the art review in rheumatology. Part 1: Current controversies and issues in the development of musculoskeletal ultrasound in rheumatology. Rheumatology 43:823-828
4. Kane D, Grassi W, Sturrock R, Balint PV (2004) Musculoskeletal ultrasound-a state of the art review in rheumatology. Part 2: Clinical indications for musculoskeletal ultrasound in rheumatology. Rheumatology 43:829-838
5. Wakefield RJ, Brown A, O'Connor P et al (2003) Rheumatological ultrasound. Rheumatology 42:1001
6. Karim Z, Wakefield RJ, Conaghan PG et al (2001) The impact of ultrasonography on diagnosis and management of patients with musculoskeletal conditions. Arthritis Rheum 44:2932-2933
7. Backhaus M, Burmester GR, Gerber T et al (2001) Guidelines for musculoskeletal ultrasound in rheumatology. Ann Rheum Dis 60:641-649
8. Grassi W, Cervini C (1998) Ultrasonography in rheumatology: an evolving technique. Ann Rheum Dis 57:268-271
9. Balint P, Sturrock RD (1997) Musculoskeletal ultrasound imaging: a new diagnostic tool for the rheumatologist? Br J Rheumatol 36:1141-1142
10. Manger B, Kalden JR (1995) Joint and connective tissue ultrasonography - A rheumatologic bedside procedure? A German experience. Arthritis Rheum 38:736-742
11. McDonald DG, Leopold GR (1972) Ultrasound B scanning in the differentiation of Baker's cyst and thrombophlebitis. Br J Radiol 45:729-733
12. Grassi W, Filippucci E, Farina A (2005) Ultrasonography in osteoarthritis. Semin Arthritis Rheum 34:19-23
13. Grassi W, Lamanna G, Farina A, Cervini C (1999) Sonographic imaging of normal and osteoarthritic cartilage. Semin Arthritis Rheum 28:398-403
14. Naredo E, Cabero F, Palop MJ et al (2005) Ultrasonographic findings in knee osteoarthritis: a comparative study with clinical and radiographic assessment. Osteoarthritis Cartilage 13:568-574
15. McCune WJ, Dedrick DK, Aisen AM, MacGuire A (1990) Sonographic evaluation of osteoarthritic femoral condylar cartilage. Correlation with operative findings. Clin Orthop 254:230-235

16. Martino F, Monetti G (1993) Semeiotica ecografica delle malattie reumatiche. Piccin ed., Padova
17. Aisen AM, McCune WJ, MacGuire A et al (1984) Sonographic evaluation of the cartilage of the knee. Radiology 153:781-784
18. Martino F, Ettorre GC, Patella V et al (1993) Articular cartilage echography as a criterion of the evolution of osteoarthritis of the knee. Int J Clin Pharmacol Res 13:35-42
19. Grassi W, Filippucci E, Farina A, Cervini C (2000) Sonographic imaging of the distal phalanx. Semin Arthritis Rheum 29:379-384
20. Iagnocco A, Filippucci E, Ossandon A et al (2005) High resolution ultrasonography in detection of bone erosions in patients with hand osteoarthritis. J Rheumatol 32:2381-2383
21. Grassi W, Tittarelli E, Pirani O et al (1993) Ultrasound examination of metacarpophalangeal joints in rheumatoid arthritis. Scand J Rheumatol 22:243-247
22. Grassi W, Tittarelli E, Blasetti P et al (1995) Finger tendon involvement in rheumatoid arthritis: evaluation with high frequency sonography. Arthritis Rheum 38:786-794
23. Lund PJ, Heikal A, Maricic MJ et al (1995) Ultrasonographic imaging of the hand and wrist in rheumatoid arthritis. Skeletal Radiol 24:591-596
24. Backhaus M, Kamradt T, Sandrock D et al (1999) Arthritis of the finger joints: a comprehensive approach comparing conventional radiography, scintigraphy, ultrasound, and contrast-enhanced magnetic resonance imaging. Arthritis Rheum 42:1232-1245
25. Grassi W, Filippucci E, Farina A et al (2001) Ultrasonography in the evaluation of bone erosions. Ann Rheum Dis 60:98-103
26. Wakefield RJ, Gibbon WW, Conaghan PG et al (2000) The value of sonography in the detection of bone erosions in patients with rheumatoid arthritis: a comparison with conventional radiography. Arthritis Rheum 43:2762-2770
27. Schmidt WA (2001) Value of sonography in diagnosis of rheumatoid arthritis. Lancet 357:1056-1057
28. Szkudlarek M, Court-Payen M, Jacobsen S et al (2003) Interobserver agreement in ultrasonography of the finger and toe joints in rheumatoid arthritis. Arthritis Rheum 48:955-962
29. Szkudlarek M, Court-Payen M, Strandberg C et al (2001) power Doppler ultrasonography for assessment of synovitis in the metacarpophalangeal joints of patients with rheumatoid arthritis: a comparison with dynamic magnetic resonance imaging. Arthritis Rheum 44:2018-2023
30. Naredo E, Gamero F, Bonilla G et al (2005) Ultrasonographic assessment of inflammatory activity in rheumatoid arthritis: comparison of extended versus reduced joint evaluation. Clin Exp Rheumatol 23:881-884
31. Weidekamm C, Koller M, Weber M, Kainberger F (2003) Diagnostic value of high-resolution B-mode and doppler sonography for imaging of hand and finger joints in rheumatoid arthritis. Arthritis Rheum 48:325-333
32. Stone M, Bergin D, Whelan B et al (2001) Power Doppler ultrasound assessment of rheumatoid hand synovitis. J Rheumatol 28:1979-1982
33. Hau M, Kneitz C, Tony HP et al (2002) High resolution ultrasound detects a decrease in pannus vascularisation of small finger joints in patients with rheumatoid arthritis receiving treatment with soluble tumour necrosis factor alpha receptor (etanercept). Ann Rheum Dis 61:55-58
34. Grassi W, Filippucci E (2003) Is power Doppler sonography the new frontier in therapy monitoring? Clin Exp Rheumatol 21:424-428
35. Wakefield RJ, Brown AK, O'Connor PJ, Emery P (2003) Power Doppler sonography: improving disease activity assessment in inflammatory musculoskeletal disease. Arthritis Rheum 48:285-288
36. Grassi W, Filippucci E, Farina A, Cervini C (2000) Sonographic imaging of tendons. Arthritis Rheum 43:969-976
37. Kane D, Greaney T, Bresnihan B et al (1999) Ultrasonography in the diagnosis and management of psoriatic dactylitis. J Rheumatol 26:1746-1751
38. Olivieri I, Barozzi L, Favaro L et al (1996) Dactylitis in patients with seronegative spondylarthropathy. Assessment by ultrasonography and magnetic resonance imaging. Arthritis Rheum 39:1524-1528
39. Balint PV, Sturrock RD (2000) Inflamed retrocalcaneal bursa and Achilles tendonitis in psoriatic arthritis demonstrated by ultrasonography. Ann Rheum Dis 59:931-933
40. Balint PV, Kane D, Wilson H et al (2002) Ultrasonography of entheseal insertions in the lower limb in spondyloarthropathy. Ann Rheum Dis 61:905-910
41. Falsetti P, Frediani B, Fioravanti A et al (2003) Sonographic study of calcaneal entheses in erosive osteoarthritis, nodal osteoarthritis, rheumatoid arthritis and psoriatic arthritis. Scand J Rheumatol 32:229-234
42. Galluzzo E, Lischi DM, Taglione E et al (2000) Sonographic analysis of the ankle in patients with psoriatic arthritis. Scand J Rheumatol 29:52-55
43. D'Agostino MA, Said-Nahal R, Hacquard-Bouder C et al (2003) Assessment of peripheral enthesitis in the spondylarthropathies by ultrasonography combined with power Doppler: a cross-sectional study. Arthritis Rheum 48:523-533
44. Frediani B, Falsetti P, Storri L et al (2002) Ultrasound and clinical evaluation of quadricipital tendon enthesitis in patients with psoriatic arthritis and rheumatoid arthritis. Clin Rheumatol 21:294-298
45. Falsetti P, Frediani B, Filippou G et al (2002) Enthesitis of proximal insertion of the deltoid in the course of seronegative spondyloarthritis. An atypical enthesitis that can mime impingement syndrome. Scand J Rheumatol 31:158-162
46. Filippucci E, Ciapetti A, Grassi W (2003) Sonographic monitoring of gout. Reumatismo 55:184-186
47. Gerster JC, Landry M, Dufresne L, Meuwly JY (2002) Imaging of tophaceous gout: computed tomography provides specific images compared with magnetic resonance imaging and ultrasonography. Ann Rheum Dis 61:52-54
48. Frediani B, Filippou G, Falsetti P et al (2005) Diagnosis of calcium pyrophosphate dihydrate crystal deposition disease: ultrasonographic criteria proposed. Ann Rheum Dis 64:638-640
49. Coari G, Iagnocco A, Zoppini A (1995) Chondrocalcinosis: sonographic study of the knee. Clin Rheumatol 14:511-514

50. Sofka CM, Adler RS, Cordasco FA (2002) Ultrasound diagnosis of chondrocalcinosis in the knee. Skeletal Radiol 31:43-45

51. Foldes K (2002) Knee chondrocalcinosis: an ultrasonographic study of the hyalin cartilage. Clin Imaging 26:194-196

52. Alasaarela E, Leppilahti J, Hakala M (1998) Ultrasound and operative evaluation of arthritic shoulder joints. Ann Rheum Dis 57:357-360

53. Naredo E, Aguado P, De Miguel E et al (2002) Painful shoulder: comparison of physical examination and ultrasonographic findings. Ann Rheum Dis 61:132-136

54. Strunk J, Lange U, Kurten B et al (2003) Doppler sonographic findings in the long bicipital tendon sheath in patients with rheumatoid arthritis as compared with patients with degenerative diseases of the shoulder. Arthritis Rheum 48:1828-1832

55. van Holsbeeck MT, Kolowich PA, Eyler WR et al (1995) US depiction of partial-thickness tear of the rotator cuff. Radiology 197:443-446

56. Teefey SA, Middleton WD, Payne WT, Yamaguchi K (2005) Detection and measurement of rotator cuff tears with sonography: analysis of diagnostic errors. AJR Am J Roentgenol 184:1768-1773

57. Bude RO, Nesbitt SD, Adler RS, Rubenfire M (1998) Sonographic detection of xanthomas in normal-sized Achilles' tendons of individuals with heterozygous familial hypercholesterolemia. AJR Am J Roentgenol 170:621-625

58. Iagnocco A, Ossandon A, Coari G et al (2004) Wrist joint involvement in systemic lupus erythematosus. An ultrasonographic study. Clin Exp Rheumatol 22:621-624

59. Ihn H, Shimozuma M, Fujmoto M et al (1995) Ultrasound measurement of skin thickness in systemic sclerosis. Br J Rheumatol 34:535-538

60. Bravo SM, Winalski CS, Weissman BN (1996) Pigmented villonodular synovitis. Radiol Clin North Am 34:311-326

61. Yang PY, Wang CL, Wu CT et al (1998) Sonography of pigmented villonodular synovitis in the ankle joint. J Clin Ultrasound 26:166-170

62. Strouse PJ, DiPietro MA, Adler RS (1998) Pediatric hip effusions: evaluation with power Doppler sonography. Radiology 206:731-735

63. Marchal GJ, Van Holsbeeck MT, Raes M et al (1987) Transient synovitis of the hip in children: role of US. Radiology 162:825-828

64. Gordon JE, Huang M, Dobbs M et al (2002) Causes of false-negative ultrasound scans in the diagnosis of septic arthritis of the hip in children. J Pediatr Orthop 22:312-316

65. Bagnolesi P, Campassi C, Cilotti A et al (1993) Artropatia emofilica: ecografia e radiologia. La radiologia medica 85:28-33

66. Klukowska A, Czyrny Z, Laguna P et al (2001) Correlation between clinical, radiological and ultrasonographical image of knee joints in children with hemophilia. Haemophilia 7:286-292

67. Lanzillo B, Pappone N, Crisci C et al (1998) Subclinical peripheral nerve involvement in patients with rheumatoid arthritis. Arthritis Rheum 41:1196-1202

68. Rosenbaum R (2001) Neuromuscular complications of connective tissue diseases. Muscle Nerve 24:154-169

69. Said G, Lacroix C (2005) Primary and secondary vasculitis neuropathy. J Neurol 252:633-641

70. Nadkar MY, Agarwal R, Samant RS et al (2001) Neuropathy in rheumatoid arthritis. J Assoc Physicians India 49:217-220

71. Sivri A, Guler-Uysal F (1998) The electroneurophysiological evaluation of rheumatoid arthritis patients. Clin Rheumatol 17:416-418

72. Buchberger W, Judmaier W, Birbamer G et al (1992) Carpal tunnel syndrome: diagnosis with high-resolution sonography. AJR 159:793-798

73. Chen P, Maklad N, Redwine M et al (1997) Dynamic high-resolution sonography of the carpal tunnel. AJR 168:533-537

74. Duncan I, Sullivan P, Lomas F (1999) Sonography in the diagnosis of carpal tunnel syndrome. AJR 173:681-683

75. Altinok T, Baysal O, Karakas HM et al (2004) Ultrasonographic assessment of mild and moderate idiopathic carpal tunnel syndrome. Clin Radiology 59:916-925

76. El-Karabaty H, Hetzel A, Galla TJ et al (2005) The effect of carpal tunnel release on median nerve flattening and nerve conduction. Electromyogr Clin Neurophysiol 45:223-227

77. Martinoli C, Bianchi S, Gandolfo N et al (2000) US of nerve entrapments in osteofibrous tunnels of the upper and lower limbs. Radiographics 20:199-217

78. Grassi W, Farina A, Filippucci E et al (2002) Intralesional therapy in carpal tunnel syndrome: a sonographic-guided approach. Clin Exp Rheumatol 20:73-76

79. Chiou HJ, Chou YH, Cheng SP et al (1998) Cubital tunnel syndrome: diagnosis by high-resolution ultrasonography. J Ultrasound Med 17:643-648

80. Jacob D, Creteur V, Courthaliac C et al (2004) Sonoanatomy of the ulnar nerve in the cubital tunnel: a multicentre study by the GEL. Eur Radiol 14:1770-1773

81. Spinner RJ, Morgenlander JC, Nunley JA (2000) Ulnar nerve function following total elbow arthroplasty: a prospective study comparing preoperative and postoperative clinical and electrophysiological evaluation in patients with rheumatoid arthritis. J Hand Surg 25:360-364

82. Pellman E, Kumari S, Greenwald R (1986) Rheumatoid iliopsoas bursitis presenting as unilateral leg edema. J Rheumatol 13:197-200

83. Bianchi S, Martinoli C, Keller A et al (2002) Giant iliopsoas bursitis: ultrasound findings with MRI correlations. J Clin Ultrasound 30: 437-441

84. Yoon TR, Song EK, Chung JY et al (2000) Femoral neuropathy caused by enlarged iliopsoas bursa associated with osteonecrosis of femoral head: a case report. Acta Orthop Scand 71:322-324

85. Mahlfeld K, Kayser R, Franke J (2004) Ultrasonographic visualization of a Baker-cyst as cause of a peroneal nerve palsy in a patient with rheumatoid arthritis. Unfallchirurg 107:429-432

86. Lee D, Dauphinée DM (2005) Morphological and functional changes in the diabetic peripheral nerve using diagnostic ultrasound and neurosensory testing to select candidates for nerve decompression J Am Podiatr Med Assoc 95:433-437

87. Lane NE, Michel B, Bjorkengren A et al (1993) The risk of osteoarthritis with running and aging: a 5-year longitudinal study. J Rheumatol 20:461-468

88. Koulouris G, Connell D (2005) Hamstring muscle complex: an imaging review. Radiographics 25:571-586
89. Connell DA, Schneider-Kolsky ME, Hoving JL et al (2004) Longitudinal study comparing sonographic and MRI assessments of acute and healing hamstring injuries. AJR Am J Roentgenol 183:975-984
90. Ulreich N, Kainberger F, Huber W, Nehrer S (2002) Achilles tendon and sports. Radiologe 42:811-817
91. Fredberg U, Bolvig L (2002) Significance of ultrasonographically detected asymptomatic tendinosis in the patellar and achilles tendons of elite soccer players: a longitudinal study. Am J Sports Med 30:488-491
92. Fredberg U, Bolvig L, Pfeiffer-Jensen M et al (2004) Ultrasonography as a tool for diagnosis, guidance of local steroid injection and, together with pressure algometry, monitoring of the treatment of athletes with chronic jumper's knee and Achilles tendinitis: a randomized, double-blind, placebo-controlled study. Scand J Rheumatol 33:94-101
93. Peers KH, Brys PP, Lysens RJ (2003) Correlation between power Doppler ultrasonography and clinical severity in Achilles tendinopathy. Int Orthop 27:180-183
94. Reiter M, Ulreich N, Dirisamer A et al (2004) Colour and power Doppler sonography in symptomatic Achilles tendon disease. Int J Sports Med 25:301-305
95. Richards PJ, Win T, Jones PW (2005) The distribution of microvascular response in Achilles tendonopathy assessed by colour and power Doppler. Skeletal Radiol 34:336-342
96. Sabir N, Demirlenk S, Yagci B et al (2005) Clinical utility of sonography in diagnosing plantar fasciitis. J Ultrasound Med 24:1041-1048
97. Bonaldi VM, Chhem RK, Drolet R et al (1998) Iliotibial band friction syndrome: sonographic findings. J Ultrasound Med 17:257-260
98. Gisslen K, Alfredson H (2005) Neovascularisation and pain in jumper's knee: a prospective clinical and sonographic study in elite junior volleyball players. Br J Sports Med 39:423-428
99. Biundo JJ Jr, Irwin RW, Umpierre E (2001) Sports and other soft tissue injuries, tendinitis, bursitis, and occupation-related syndromes. Curr Opin Rheumatol 13:146-149
100. Gibson T (1987) Sports injuries. Baillieres Clin Rheumatol 1:583-600
101. Brasseur JL, Lucidarme O, Tardieu M et al (2004) Ultrasonographic rotator-cuff changes in veteran tennis players: the effect of hand dominance and comparison with clinical findings. Eur Radiol 14:857-864
102. Ueblacker P, Gebauer M, Ziegler M et al (2005) Sports injuries and overuse syndromes. Bundesgesundheitsblatt Gesundheitsforschung Gesundheitsschutz 48:927-938
103. Brasseur JL, Zeitoun-Eiss D (2005) Ultrasound of acute disorders of the shoulder. JBR-BTR 88:193-199
104. Bianchi S, Martinoli C, Abdelwahab IF (2005) Ultrasound of tendon tears. Part 1: general considerations and upper extremity. Skeletal Radiol 34:500-512
105. Hume PA, Reid D, Edwards T (2006) Epicondylar injury in sport: epidemiology, type, mechanisms, assessment, management and prevention. Sports Med 36:151-170
106. Silvestri E, Biggi E, Molfetta L et al (2003) Power Doppler analysis of tendon vascularization. Int J Tissue React 25:149-158
107. Maganaris CN, Narici MV, Almekinders LC, Maffulli N (2004) Biomechanics and pathophysiology of overuse tendon injuries: ideas on insertional tendinopathy. Sports Med 34:1005-1017
108. Jacobson JA (2002) Ultrasound in sports medicine. Radiol Clin North Am 40:363-386
109. Bianchi S, Poletti PA, Martinoli C (2006) Ultrasound appearance of tendon tears. Part 2: lower extremity and myotendinous tears. Skeletal Radiol 35:63-77
110. Giuffre BM, Lisle DA (2005) Tear of the distal biceps branchii tendon: a new method of ultrasound evaluation. Australas Radiol 49:404-406
111. Moosikasuwan JB, Miller TT, Burke BJ (2005) Rotator cuff tears: clinical, radiographic, and US findings. Radiographics 25:1591-1607
112. Bianchi S, Cohen M, Jacob D (2005) Tendons: traumatic lesions. J Radiol 86:1845-1857
113. Hahn P, Schmitt R, Kall S (2001) Stener lesion yes or no? Diagnosis by ultrasound. Handchir Mikrochir Plast Chir 33:46-48

Ultrasonography and therapy monitoring

US permits accurate and reliable assessment of soft tissue involvement in rheumatic disease [1-3]. High-resolution US with power Doppler equipment can detect even minimal morphostructural and perfusional changes within soft tissues [4-14], and may offer additional information for disease activity monitoring [15-24] (Figs. 6.1-6.6).

Some preliminary investigations suggest that power Doppler US could be successfully incorporated into drug therapy monitoring in patients with

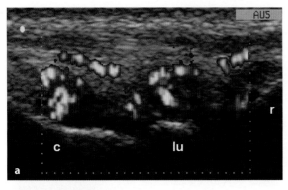
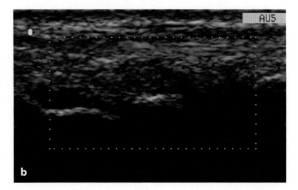

Fig. 6.1 a, b

Rheumatoid arthritis. **a** Baseline US examination with a longitudinal dorsal scan of the wrist joint. An intra-articular injection of triamcinolone acetonide (30 mg) was performed under US guidance. **b** Two weeks after the injection, follow-up US examination detected a dramatic decrease in both joint cavity widening and intra-articular power Doppler signals. *c* = capitate bone; *lu* = lunate bone; *r* = radius

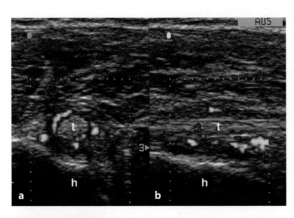
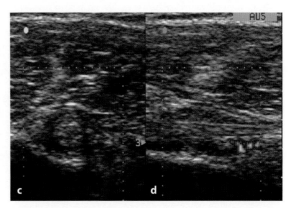

Fig. 6.2 a-d

Rheumatoid arthritis. Baseline US examination on transverse (**a**) and longitudinal (**b**) anterior scans of the shoulder showing active tenosynovitis of the long head of biceps tendon (*t*). An injection of triamcinolone acetonide (30 mg) was performed under US guidance within the tendon sheath. **c, d** Two weeks after the injection, follow-up US examination detected a marked reduction of power Doppler signal. *h* = bicipital groove

synovitis, but further verification in larger numbers of patients is required.

Power Doppler US with high-resolution probes can demonstrate a raised blood volume both around and within joints and tendons. These changes occur in patients with synovitis because of increased perfusion and/or angiogenesis. Thus, power Doppler US could play an interesting role in therapy monitoring because of its safety, repeatability and low operative cost.

In patients with active synovitis, power Doppler signal can be identified with appropriate setting of the US equipment. Lack of signal within and under the bone profile and a "pulse repetition frequency" of 700-1000 Hz appear to be the best compromise between the sensitivity and the specificity of power Doppler.

Several limitations of power Doppler US have to be kept in mind. Images are operator-dependent and machine-dependent. Artifacts are com-

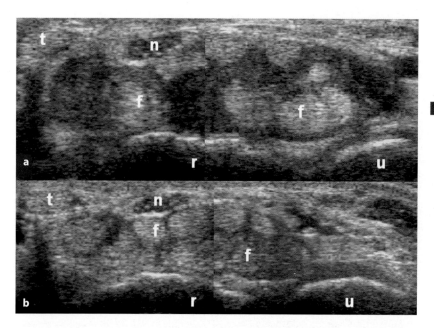

Fig. 6.3 a, b

Rheumatoid arthritis. Carpal tunnel syndrome due to proliferative tenosynovitis of the finger flexor tendons (*f*). **a** Baseline US examination on transverse scan showing marked tendon sheath widening. An injection of triamcinolone acetonide (30 mg) was performed under US guidance within the tendon sheath. **b** Two weeks after the injection, follow-up US examination showed no signs of tenosynovitis. *r* = radius; *u* = ulna; *n* = median nerve; *t* = flexor carpi radialis tendon

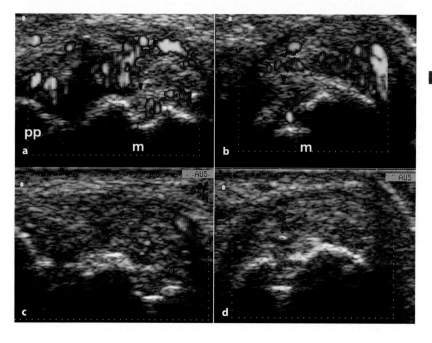

Fig. 6.4 a-d

A 72-year-old man presented with rheumatoid arthritis and active synovitis of the second metacarpophalangeal joint of the dominant hand. **a, b** Baseline US examination revealed increased intra-articular perfusion with synovial proliferation localized both around and inside an area of eroded bone at the metacarpal head. **c, d** After 3 months of treatment with intramuscular methotrexate (10 mg per week), pain improved (visual analog scale (VAS) score reduced from 9 to 0) and the intra-articular power Doppler signal almost disappeared. *m* = metacarpal head; *pp* = proximal phalanx

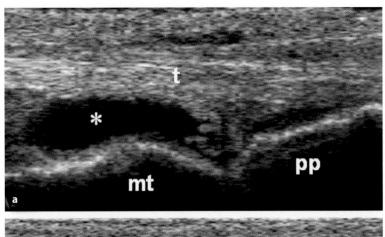

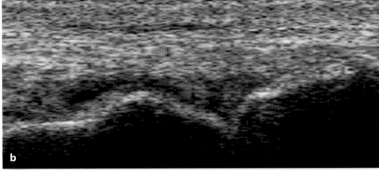

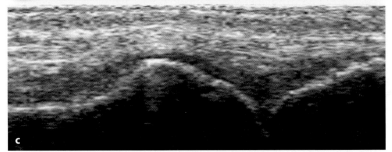

Fig. 6.5 a-c

A 48-year-old man presented with an acute attack of gout involving the first metatarsophalangeal joint of the left foot. US monitoring of acute gout on longitudinal dorsal view within 24 hours of the onset of synovitis (**a**) and one (**b**) and two (**c**) weeks after the baseline examination. *mt* = metatarsal head; *pp* = proximal phalanx; *t* = extensor tendon; * = synovial fluid

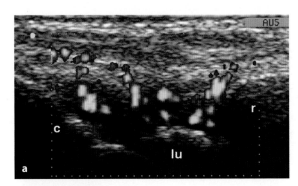

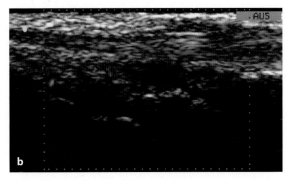

Fig. 6.6 a, b

Rheumatoid arthritis. **a** Baseline US examination on longitudinal dorsal scan of the wrist joint. **b** Six weeks after receiving 40 mg adalimumab administered subcutaneously fortnightly, a marked reduction in both joint cavity widening and intra-articular power Doppler signal was detected. *c* = capitate bone; *lu* = lunate bone; *r* = radius

mon and sometimes they can lead to misinterpretation [25, 26].

In spite of these limitations, power Doppler US is increasingly being regarded as an exciting research tool in the field of therapy-monitoring of rheumatic diseases [15]. Key points for future investigation include the definition of standardized examination protocols (scanning technique, position of the patient and setting of the machine) and a validated quantification of power Doppler findings.

References

1. Grassi W, Cervini C (1998) Ultrasonography in rheumatology: an evolving technique. Ann Rheum Dis 57:268-271
2. Grassi W, Salaffi F, Filippucci E (2005) Ultrasound in rheumatology. Best Pract Res Clin Rheumatol 19:467-485
3. Kane D, Grassi W, Sturrock R, Balint PV (2004) Musculoskeletal ultrasound - a state of the art review in rheumatology. Part 2: Clinical indications for musculoskeletal ultrasound in rheumatology. Rheumatology 43:829-838
4. Wakefield RJ, Brown AK, O'Connor PJ, Emery P (2003) Power Doppler sonography: improving disease activity assessment in inflammatory musculoskeletal disease. Arthritis Rheum 48:285-288
5. Hau M, Schultz H, Tony HP et al (1999) Evaluation of pannus and vascularization of the metacarpophalangeal and proximal interphalangeal joints in rheumatoid arthritis by high-resolution ultrasound (multidimensional linear array). Ann Rheum Dis 42:2303-2308
6. Rubin JM, Bude RO, Carson PL et al (1994) Power Doppler: a potentially useful alternative to mean-frequency based colour Doppler sonography. Radiology 190:853-856
7. Martinoli C, Pretolesi F, Crespi G et al (1998) Power Doppler sonography: clinical applications. Eur J Radiol 27:S133-S140
8. Newman JS, Adler RS, Bude RO, Rubin JM (1994) Detection of soft-tissue hyperemia: value of power Doppler sonography. AJR Am J Roentgenol 163:385-389
9. Breidahl WH, Newman JS, Toljanovic MS, Adler RS (1996) Power Doppler sonography in the assessment of musculoskeletal fluid collections. Am J Roentgenol 166:1443-1446
10. Walther M, Harms H, Krenn V et al (2001) Correlation of power Doppler sonography with vascularity of the synovial tissue of the knee joint in patients with osteoarthritis and rheumatoid arthritis. Arthritis Rheum 44:331-338
11. Schmidt WA, Volker L, Zacher J et al (2000) Colour Doppler ultrasonography to detect pannus in knee joint synovitis. Clin Exp Rheumatol 18:439-444
12. Szkudlarek M, Court-Payen M, Strandberg C et al (2001) Power Doppler sonography for assessment of synovitis in the metacarpophalangeal joints of patients with rheumatoid arthritis: a comparison with dynamic magnetic resonance imaging. Arthritis Rheum 44:2018-2023
13. Qvistgaard E, Rogind H, Torp-Pederson S et al (2001) Quantitative ultrasonography in rheumatoid arthritis: evaluation of inflammation by Doppler technique. Ann Rheum Dis 60:690-693
14. Carotti M, Salaffi F, Manganelli P et al (2002) Power Doppler sonography in the assessment of synovial tissue of the knee joint in rheumatoid arthritis: a preliminary experience. Ann Rheum Dis 61:877-882
15. Grassi W, Filippucci E (2003) Is power Doppler sonography the new frontier in therapy monitoring? Clin Exp Rheumatol 21:424-428
16. Newman J, Laing T, McCarthy C, Adler RS (1996) Power Doppler sonography of synovitis: assessment of therapeutic response-preliminary observations. Radiology 198:582-584
17. Stone M, Bergin D, Whelan B et al (2001) Power Doppler ultrasound assessment of rheumatoid hand synovitis. J Rheumatol 28:1979-1982
18. Hau M, Kneitz C, Tony HP et al (2002) High resolution ultrasound detects a decrease in pannus vascularisation of small finger joints in patients with rheumatoid arthritis receiving treatment with soluble tumour necrosis factor alpha receptor (etanercept). Ann Rheum Dis 61:55-58
19. Ribbens C, Andre B, Marcelis S et al (2003) Rheumatoid hand joint synovitis: gray-scale and power Doppler US quantifications following anti-tumor necrosis factor-alpha treatment: pilot study. Radiology 229:562-569
20. Terslev L, Torp-Pedersen S, Qvistgaard E et al (2003) Effects of treatment with etanercept (Enbrel, TNRF:Fc) on rheumatoid arthritis evaluated by Doppler ultrasonography. Ann Rheum Dis 62:178-181
21. Filippucci E, Farina A, Carotti M et al (2004) Grey scale and power Doppler sonographic changes induced by intra-articular steroid injection treatment. Ann Rheum Dis 63:740-743
22. Taylor PC, Steuer A, Gruber J et al (2004) Comparison of ultrasonographic assessment of synovitis and joint vascularity with radiographic evaluation in a randomized, placebo-controlled study of infliximab therapy in early rheumatoid arthritis. Arthritis Rheum 50:1107-1116
23. Taylor PC, Steuer A, Gruber J et al (2006) Ultrasonographic and radiographic results from a two-year controlled trial of immediate or one-year-delayed addition of infliximab to ongoing methotrexate therapy in patients with erosive early rheumatoid arthritis. Arthritis Rheum 54:47-53
24. Filippucci E, Iagnocco A, Salaffi F et al (2006) Power Doppler sonography monitoring of synovial perfusion at wrist joint in rheumatoid patients treated with adalimumab. Ann Rheum Dis (in press)
25. Cardinal E, Lafortune M, Burns P (1996) Power Doppler US in synovitis: reality or artifact? Radiology 200:868-869
26. Kamaya A, Tuthill T, Rubin JM (2003) Twinkling artifact on color Doppler sonography: dependence on machine parameters and underlying cause. AJR Am J Roentgenol 180:215-222

Ultrasound-guided procedures

Needle aspiration of synovial fluid and intra-lesional injection of various compounds are very common procedures in rheumatological practice. Local steroid injection, in particular, is relatively simple and cost-effective and may be alternative or adjunctive to systemic drug therapy in several rheumatological conditions [1-5]. Both efficacy and side effects of the injection depend on the correct placement of the tip of the needle inside or around the lesion. Particular attention must be taken to avoid direct needle contact with nerves, tendons, articular cartilage and blood vessels [6]. Intra-articular and intra-lesional therapy is usually performed using palpation and bony landmarks for guidance. Conventional blind interventional procedures may be particularly problematic when a small and/or deep target has to be reached, or when an injection has to be carried out into a dry joint.

It has been reported that 50% of conventional joint injections are placed incorrectly [7-8].

US guidance during such procedures may minimize both the difficulty and margin for error during intra-lesional therapy. This approach is, however, still very limited in rheumatological practice.

US-guided injections can be performed using the method where the skin surface is marked after the detection of the most appropriate entrance point and the measurement of the depth of the target area, or under direct visualization of needle placement during real-time scanning [1, 2].

US-guided injection under direct visualization should be performed according to the following principles:

1. Baseline US assessment to explore the target area and evaluate the indication for the planned injection therapy.
2. Definition of the best US window to optimize visualization of needle placement within the target area.
3. Antiseptic swabbing of both the injection site and the surface of the probe.
4. Placement of a thin layer of sterile gel on the skin of the patient.
5. Continuous monitoring of the needle progression within the soft tissues on the screen with particular attention to the tip of the needle, which is placed within the target area.
6. Visualization of the steroid suspension during and after the injection (Fig. 7.1).

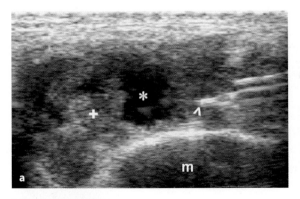
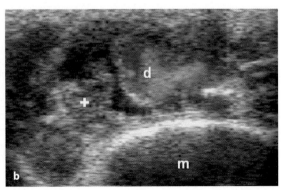

Fig. 7.1 a, b

Rheumatoid arthritis. US-guided injection of triamcinolone acetonide (5 mg) into a metacarpophalangeal joint with proliferative synovitis. **a** Placement of the tip of the needle (*arrowhead*) in the target area. **b** Visualization of the steroid suspension (*d*) during the injection. *m* = metacarpal head; * = synovial fluid; + = synovial proliferation

On longitudinal scans, when the needle is perpendicular to the US beam it appears as a sharply defined echoic band with strong posterior reverberations. On transverse scan, the needle appears as a small hyperechoic round spot that can be easily identified by dynamic assessment (fine movements of the syringe).

Confirmation of the needle's correct positioning can be obtained by direct observation by injecting air or under power Doppler control (the injected fluid is visualized as a patch of color).

Needle placement is quick and easy to perform when marked distension of the joint cavity is present. Optimal visualization of the needle depends on the correct alignment between the needle and ultrasound beam. Accurate positioning of the probe is critical to obtain a clearly defined image both of the needle and the target site (Fig. 7.2).

Local injection therapy has a well-established role in patients with tenosynovitis.

The cost/benefit ratio largely depends on the correct placement of the needle into the widened tendon sheath. An experienced rheumatologist should be able to perform a safe and accurate intra-lesional injection in most patients with tenosynovitis. The main problem is taking care to avoid contact between the tip of the needle and the tendon (Fig. 7.3).

The conventional blind approach to intra-lesional injection cannot avoid the theoretical risk of causing damage to tendons and surrounding structures.

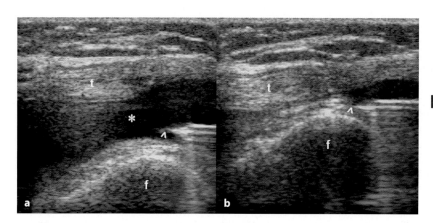

Fig. 7.2 a, b

Joint effusion in knee osteoarthritis. US-guided aspiration using a supra-patellar transverse scan with the knee extended. **a, b** Different steps during synovial fluid (*) aspiration. The *arrowhead* indicates the tip of the needle. *f* = femur; *t* = quadriceps tendon

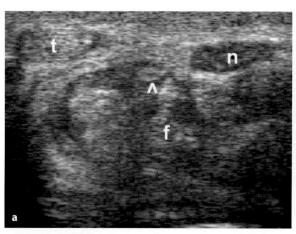
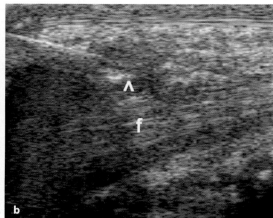

Fig. 7.3 a, b

Carpal tunnel syndrome due to rheumatoid tenosynovitis of the finger flexor tendons. Position of the tip of the needle is accurately visualized both on transverse (**a**) and longitudinal (**b**) scans. *arrowhead* = tip of the needle; *f* = finger flexor tendons; *n* = median nerve; *t* = flexor carpi radialis tendon

The injection of steroids within a widened tendon sheath under US control appears to be very effective in minimizing this risk. The progression of the needle can be accurately controlled "step by step" on the monitor until the tip of the needle is properly placed within the tendon sheath.

Bursitis is a very common problem in rheumatological practice. Injection of steroid is an effective and safe procedure in non-responders to other conservative therapeutic options, including rest, local application of ice and anti-inflammatory medication. The US approach to patients with suspected bursitis serves three purposes: firstly, confirmation of the diagnosis; secondly, aspiration of synovial fluid for microscopic examination and thirdly, correct placement of the needle for steroid injection.

US is very useful for the detection of popliteal cysts and for careful assessment of their content. Once the inner structure of the cyst is established, it is possible to define an appropriate therapeutic approach that depends on the cyst characteristics. Needle aspiration of synovial fluid and steroid injection within a popliteal cyst under US control are indicated especially in patients with large cysts due to a valve effect of the synovial tissue. US control is critical to avoid puncture wounds of nerves and/or blood vessels and to ensure the correct position of the tip of the needle especially in patients with loculated cysts.

References

1. Koski JM (2000) Ultrasound guided injections in rheumatology. J Rheumatol 27:2131-2138
2. Grassi W, Farina A, Filippucci E, Cervini C (2001) Sonographically guided procedures in rheumatology. Semin Arthritis Rheum 30:347-353
3. Grassi W, Farina A, Filippucci E, Cervini C (2002) Intralesional therapy in carpal tunnel syndrome: a sonographic-guided approach. Clin Exp Reumatol 20:73-76
4. Qvistgaard E, Kristoffersen H, Terslev L et al (2001) Guidance by ultrasound of intra-articular injections in the knee and hip joints. Osteoarthritis Cartilage 9:512-517
5. Balint PV, Kane D, Sturrock RD (2001) Modern patient management in rheumatology: interventional musculoskeletal ultrasonography. Osteoarthritis Cartilage 9:509-511
6. Kumar N, Newmon RJ (1999) Complications of intra- and peri-articular steroid injections. Br J Gen Pract 49:465-466
7. Jones A, Regan M, Ledingham J et al (1993) Importance of placement of intra-articular steroid injections. Br Med J 307:1329-1330
8. Eustace JA, Brophy DP, Gibney RP et al (1997) Comparison of the accuracy of steroid placement with clinical outcome in patients with shoulder symptoms. Ann Rheum Dis 56:59-63